"An important co... ...p...
of inequalities from COVID itself, the
lockdown and the economic impacts."
James Dunn, McMaster University

"A brilliant dissection of the COVID-19 pandemic.
The authors paint a picture of its unequal health, economic and
social impacts and conclude with hopes for a
brighter future."
**Fran Baum, Southgate Institute for Health, Society and
Equity, Flinders University**

"This vital book doesn't just show the inequality of COVID's
consequences, it demonstrates how inequalities have undermined
the response. It exposes them as political choices, and sets out the
policies to beat inequality, COVID, and the pandemics to come."
**Ben Phillips, author of *How to Fight Inequality* and
advisor to the United Nations**

"This book provides a clear and thorough account of how
COVID-19 has exposed and is exacerbating deep-seated
inequalities in our societies, and how this is impacting on what
citizens value most, their health. An important read."
Caroline Costongs, EuroHealthNet

"Stands out not only for its unflinching analysis of COVID-19's
syndemic layering of inequalities but for how this embodies a
pathological political economy that must be transformed."
Ronald Labonté, University of Ottawa

CLARE BAMBRA, JULIA LYNCH,
KATHERINE E. SMITH
WITH A FOREWORD BY
PROFESSOR KATE PICKETT

THE UNEQUAL
PANDEMIC

COVID-19 and Health Inequalities

P

First published in Great Britain in 2021 by

Policy Press, an imprint of
Bristol University Press
University of Bristol
1–9 Old Park Hill
Bristol
BS2 8BB
UK
t: +44 (0)117 954 5940
e: bup-info@bristol.ac.uk

Details of international sales and distribution partners are available at
policy.bristoluniversitypress.co.uk

© Bristol University Press 2021

British Library Cataloguing in Publication Data
A catalogue record for this book is available from the British Library

ISBN 978-1-4473-6123-7 paperback
ISBN 978-1-4473-6125-1 ePdf
ISBN 978-1-4473-6124-4 ePub

Cover design by Dave Worth
Front cover image: Getty / Angela Weiss

Contents

List of figures and tables

Figures

Tables

About the authors

Clare Bambra is Professor of Public Health, Population Health Sciences Institute, Faculty of Medical Sciences, Newcastle University, UK. She is an interdisciplinary social scientist working at the interface of public health, health politics and policy, health geography and social epidemiology. Her mixed-methods research focuses on understanding and reducing health inequalities. She has published extensively including several books: *Work, Worklessness and the Political Economy of Health* (Oxford University Press, 2011), *How Politics Makes Us Sick – Neoliberal Epidemics* (Palgrave Macmillan, 2015), *Health Divides: Where You Live Can Kill You* (2016, Policy Press), *Health in Hard Times* (2019, Policy Press); with Katherine E. Smith, a British Medical Association award-winning edited collection, *Health Inequalities: Critical Perspectives* (Oxford University Press, 2015); and with Julia Lynch, *Interests, Inequalities and the Politics of Ageing and Health* (Cambridge University Press, 2021).
Twitter @ProfBambra

Julia Lynch is Professor of Political Science, Department of Political Science, at the University of Pennsylvania, US. Her research focuses on the politics of inequality, public health and social policy in rich democracies, particularly the countries of western Europe. She has special interests in comparative health policy and the politics of health inequalities; comparative political economy of western Europe; southern European politics; and the politics of ageing. She is the editor of *Socio-Economic Review* and serves on the editorial boards of *Perspectives in Politics, Comparative Political Studies, Polity, Journal of European Social Policy* and *Journal of Health Politics, Policy and Law*. She has published widely including: *Regimes of Inequality: The Political Economy of Health and Wealth* (Cambridge University Press, 2020), *Age in the Welfare State: The Origins of Social Spending on Pensioners, Workers, and Children* (Cambridge University Press, 2006), and with Clare Bambra, *Interests, Inequalities and the Politics of Ageing and Health* (Cambridge University Press, 2021). Twitter @juliaflynch

Katherine E. Smith is Professor of Public Health Policy, Department of Social Policy at the University of Strathclyde, UK. Her principal research interests concern understanding who shapes the policies impacting on public health and how. She has a long track record of studying the interplay between evidence, expertise and policy, and of critically analysing policy responses to public health crises (especially health inequalities). Her publications include *Beyond Evidence-Based Public Health Policy: The Interplay of Ideas* (Palgrave Macmillan, 2013), and a British Medical Association award-winning edited collection, with Clare Bambra, *Health Inequalities: Critical Perspectives* (Oxford University Press, 2015). She is co-editor-in-chief of the Policy Press journal *Evidence & Policy*.
Twitter @ProfKatSmith

Acknowledgements

We would like to thank Victoria Morgan of Newcastle University for administrative support.

We would like to acknowledge the following grant funding that supported this book: Clare Bambra is a senior investigator in *CHAIN: Centre for Global Health Inequalities Research* (Norwegian Research Council 288638), *NIHR ARC North East and North Cumbria* (NIHR200173), the *NIHR School of Public Health Research* (PD-SPH-2015) and *Fuse: the Centre for Translational Research in Public Health*. She is also funded by a *Health Foundation COVID-19 grant* (2211473) and *SIPHER: Systems Science in Public Health and Health Economics Research Consortium* (MR/S037578/1). Katherine E. Smith is a senior investigator in *SIPHER* (MR/S037578/1) and a member of the *SPECTRUM Consortium* (MR/S037519/1). The *SIPHER* and *SPECTRUM* consortiums are funded by the UK Prevention Research Partnership Consortium. UKPRP is an initiative funded by the UK Research and Innovation Councils, the Department of Health and Social Care (England) and the UK devolved administrations, and leading health research charities. The views expressed in this publication are those of the authors and do not necessarily reflect those of the funders.

Foreword

I am writing this during the short dark days between Christmas and New Year at the end of a strange and difficult year, a year in which practitioners of my discipline, epidemiologists, have come to unexpected prominence and recognition. Epidemiology is the study and analysis of the distribution, patterns and determinants of health, disease and wellbeing in populations (rather than individuals). The word derives from the Greek 'epi': on or upon, and 'demos': the people, so in essence, 'what befalls the people'. What has befallen us during 2020 has often been described as an unprecedented global challenge, and yet human history has, time and again, been plagued by epidemics and pandemics – from the Antonine Plague in 165 AD (thought to be smallpox), through the Black Death in 1350, the devastation of the indigenous populations of the Americas after they came into contact with Europeans, the Great Plague of London in 1665, the 1918 Spanish flu and the worldwide ravages of HIV/AIDS since the 1980s, just to name a few.

Our science of epidemiology, as it seeks to understand both the causes and the consequences of states of health and disease, underpins practice and action that promotes and protects the people's wellbeing. And historically our science has never been confined to the laboratory or the hospital; it has been hand-in-glove and inextricably intertwined with social justice and human rights campaigning, from the earliest interventions to improve sanitation and protect child labourers in the squalid cities of the Industrial Revolution to the high-level policy that will determine the likelihood of equitable distribution of COVID-19 vaccinations across the globe. Our epidemiological science and our public health practice are nothing if they do not reach all the people of the world, including all those who are 'othered', such as the poor, the marginalised and the dispossessed.

Throughout 2020 we have been told repeatedly by political leaders that they are 'following the science'. This is a welcome pivot from being told that 'the people of this country have had enough of experts', even if the shift is to some extent an attempt to evade responsibility and accountability for the suffering caused by the responses to the COVID-19 pandemic, including lockdowns and closures of schools and workplaces. But why haven't political leaders always followed the science? Epidemiologists and public health specialists have spent decades trying to draw attention to the vast inequalities in health that fracture our societal wellbeing and prosperity. From the Black Report of 1980 through the Marmot Review of 2010 and beyond, there has been a consistent message that action is needed, consistent data on the scale of the problem, and a consistent consensus on what needs to be done. If our political leaders had been paying attention to the science of epidemiology and public health before the pandemic, we would not have been so fragile and fewer of us would have died during it.

Our discipline has matured with time. It began with the recognition of germ theory and the need for population-based measures to ensure adequate food, shelter and clean water to prevent and ameliorate infectious disease; later it focused more on chronic conditions – cancer, diabetes, heart disease – and the ways in which individual behaviours shaped health. Its most recent flourishing has been in the recognition that the quality of relationships between us is fundamental to health. Friendship is as protective of our health as smoking is bad for it. Loneliness can kill. Hope and optimism can heal your (physical) heart as well as your soul. Dignity and a sense of being treated fairly can save your life. Think about all these 'social determinants' of health: none of them are distributed equally, and all of them are intertwined. The authors of this book understand what has befallen us this year; they know what shaped the public's health before the pandemic, and how unequally the pandemic has been experienced; even more importantly, they know what needs to be done to care for and repair both the health of the people and the body politic.

Professor Kate Pickett
York, UK, 28 December 2020

Preface

In 1931 Edgar Sydenstricker identified inequalities in the 1918 Spanish flu epidemic, reporting a significantly higher incidence among the working classes.[1] This challenged the widely-held popular, political and scientific consensus of the time that claimed 'the flu hit the rich and the poor alike'. In the 2020 COVID-19 pandemic, there have been parallel claims made by politicians and the media: that we are 'all in it together' and that the COVID-19 virus 'does not discriminate'.

This book aims to dispel the emerging myth of COVID-19 as an 'equality of opportunity' disease, by outlining how, just as 100 years ago, the pandemic is experienced unequally across society. COVID-19 and inequality are a syndemic: a perfect storm. Drawing on international data and accounts, the book will argue that the pandemic is unequal in four ways:

The pandemic kills unequally: COVID-19 deaths are twice as high in the most deprived neighbourhoods of England as in the most affluent; infection rates are higher in the more deprived regions, such as the northeast of England, and in urban compared to rural areas. There are also significant inequalities by ethnicity and race, with the mortality of ethnic minorities in the UK considerably higher than expected, and the death rates of Black Americans in US cities such as Chicago are far higher than for their White counterparts. This is because of the interaction of the pandemic with existing social, economic and health inequalities.

The pandemic is experienced unequally: the COVID-19 lockdowns have resulted in a significant increase in social isolation and confinement within the home and immediate neighbourhood for an average of 10–12 weeks. The social and economic experiences of this lockdown are unequal as lower-income workers are more likely to experience job and income loss, live in higher-risk urban and overcrowded environments, and have higher exposure to the virus by occupying key worker roles.

The pandemic impoverishes unequally: COVID-19 and the lockdowns have resulted in an unprecedented shock to the economy, with widespread predictions of the worst recession for 300 years. This economic devastation will result in job losses, wage reductions, higher debt, and more poverty, as well as increases in the 'deaths of despair'. However, the social and geographical distribution of these economic impacts will be unequal, with low-income workers, women and ethnic minorities bearing the brunt.

The pandemic inequalities are political: the unequal impacts of COVID-19 were not inevitable: the pandemic was a predictable event and the unequal effects could have been mitigated or avoided through better preparation. The original inequalities leading to these unequal impacts were a result of prior political choices, and policymakers could choose whether to address the unequal impacts of the pandemic, or not. Governments responded differently, and those with higher rates of social inequality and less generous social security systems had a more unequal pandemic.

COVID-19 is a **syndemic of infectious disease and inequalities**. It has killed unequally, been experienced unequally and will impoverish unequally. These health inequalities, before, during and after the pandemic are a political choice – with governments effectively choosing who gets to live and who gets to die. We need to learn from COVID-19 quickly to prevent inequality growing and to reduce health inequalities in the future.

ONE

Introduction: perfect storm

Perfect storm: a particularly violent storm arising from a rare combination of negative factors.[1]

COVID-19: the unequal pandemic

In December 2019, the first cases of an unusual 'pneumonia' were documented in the Chinese city of Wuhan. The novel disease, which seems to have jumped from an animal population into humans, was later named 'SARS-CoV-2' or 'COVID-19' (coronavirus disease 2019). The entire city of Wuhan, with a population over 11 million, was put under stringent quarantine by the Chinese government, with the lockdown eventually lasting 76 days. But by January 2020, the disease had spread to the US, Europe and the UK, and at the end of the month the World Health Organization (WHO) declared COVID-19 a 'public health emergency of international concern'. By February, the first death attributed to coronavirus was reported outside of China, in the Philippines, and France announced the first coronavirus death in Europe. By the end of February, COVID-19 cases had been reported across all world regions and by mid-March, the epicenter of the COVID-19 pandemic had moved from China to Europe. By the end of March countries as varied as the UK, India, France and Norway had introduced emergency measures (social distancing and lockdowns) to try and contain the virus.[2] The COVID-19 pandemic had begun.

COVID-19 is now a global phenomenon, affecting all parts of the world and all parts of society, radically altering how we live and interact. Everyone, from all walks of life, has been affected by the pandemic. But, as this book will show, some people have been – and will be – far more affected than others: COVID-19 is an unequal pandemic.

High-profile early cases of the virus included powerful and wealthy individuals such as Prince Charles, UK prime minister Boris Johnson, and Hollywood actor Tom Hanks. This gave the impression, often reinforced in claims made by politicians and the media, that when it came to COVID-19 we are 'all in it together', and that the COVID-19 virus 'does not discriminate'. In one sense, this is true: the virus, once contracted, can bring serious illness or death no matter how wealthy or powerful the 'host'.

But wealth and power *do* provide layers of protection from the disease: they make it less likely that a person will be exposed to the virus, and less likely that they will suffer its worst effects (including death). And as the pandemic has developed, its fundamentally unequal nature has become more clear: infection rates are higher in more deprived regions, among people with low incomes, and in urban compared to rural areas; and COVID-19 deaths are twice as high in the most deprived neighbourhoods as in the most affluent. There are even more stark inequalities by ethnicity and race, with minority ethnic groups in countries like England, Canada and the US experiencing death rates that are up to three times as high as their White majority counterparts. Emergency measures taken to contain the virus, including lockdowns, have also impacted people unequally, and the growing economic crisis created by the pandemic is already being experienced unequally. This book exposes these inequalities, examining how and why COVID-19 is an unequal pandemic.

This introductory chapter sets out our main argument: the COVID-19 pandemic is not only experienced unequally, but is actually a *syndemic pandemic*, interacting with and exacerbated by social, economic and health inequalities – a rare combination of negative factors producing a 'perfect storm'. It describes the key concepts and metaphors used in the book, including health inequalities (health differences between social groups defined by, for example, socioeconomic status, geography, gender and race/ethnicity); the social determinants of health (how the conditions in which we live, work and age impact on our health); and the 'perfect storm' of a syndemic pandemic that has occurred as health inequalities and the social determinants of health interact with a novel virus.

Health inequalities

'Health inequality' refers to the systematic differences in health that exist between people and places, characterised by differences in socioeconomic status (SES) (for example, between income groups, levels of education, occupational background); levels of socioeconomic deprivation (for example, areas with greater or lesser economic, social and physical infrastructure); race/ethnicity (for example, between Black and White Americans); or gender. These systematic differences in health between groups in society are labelled as inequalities or inequities because they are unfair: 'As they are socially produced, they are potentially avoidable and widely considered unacceptable in a civilised society'.[3] Inequalities in health are not restricted to differences between the most privileged groups and the most disadvantaged, however. Health inequalities exist across the entire social gradient, from the most disadvantaged through the middle classes to the wealthiest and most powerful members of society.[4] The social gradient in health runs from the top to the bottom of society, which means that 'even comfortably off people somewhere in the middle tend to have poorer health than those above them'.[5]

In all high-income countries, including those as varied as the UK, the US, France and Norway, inequalities in health by socioeconomic status, levels of deprivation, and race/ethnicity are stark.[6] In the UK, for example, Londoners living in Canning Town at one end of the Jubilee tube line live seven years less on average than those living eight stops along the line in Westminster.[7] There is a 15-year gap in life expectancy between residents of the affluent Cathcart and deprived Possilpark and Ruchill neighbourhoods of Glasgow – the largest health divide in Europe.[8] Across England, the average life expectancy at birth gap between the most and least deprived areas is nine years for men and seven years for women.[9] Likewise, the gap in average healthy life expectancy is 18 years for men and around 19 years for women.[10] In the US city of New Orleans, there is a 25-year gap in life expectancy between rich and poor neighbourhoods, and in Oslo, the capital of Norway, life expectancy varies by up to eight years between districts.[11]

There are much higher rates of non-communicable chronic diseases (NCDs), including cardiovascular disease, cancer, diabetes, chronic obstructive pulmonary disease (COPD), and obesity among people living in more deprived neighbourhoods. Deaths from cardiovascular diseases in England are almost three times higher in the 20% most deprived areas compared to the 20% least deprived, and alcohol-related hospital admissions are more than twice as high among men and among women in the 20% most deprived areas compared to the 20% least deprived areas.[12] These health inequalities start very early in life, with stark inequalities in infant mortality rates between deprived and affluent neighbourhoods in England.[13] Deprived and affluent areas with such shocking differences in health outcomes can be located very near one another – indeed just a few miles apart.[14]

There are also large health inequalities between people from different socioeconomic backgrounds, regardless of where they live. People with higher occupational status (for example, professionals such as teachers or lawyers) have better health outcomes than those with lower occupational status (for example, manual workers).[15] Similarly, people with a higher income or university education have better health outcomes than those with a low income or no educational qualifications.[16]

Longstanding inequalities also exist between groups of different racial and ethnic backgrounds, despite the fact that there are no real biological differences between racial groups.[17] In the US, for example, African Americans (to take just one ethnic group as an example) are twice as likely to report having fair or poor health compared with non-Hispanic Whites.[18] Over 40% of African American adults suffer from hypertension compared with less than 30% of non-Hispanic White adults.[19] African Americans have the highest mortality rate for all cancers compared with any other racial and ethnic group.[20] There are 11 infant deaths per 1,000 live births among Black Americans. This is almost twice the national average of 5.8 infant deaths per 1,000 live births.[21] Health inequalities between American Indians and non-Hispanic Whites are even larger.[22]

The influences of socioeconomic status, place and race/ethnicity on health are experienced in combination, and we all have different aspects of our social identity (including gender) that coexist – and interact – with one another. Intersectionality is a way of looking at multiple influences on health. It focuses on how socioeconomic status, deprivation, ethnicity and gender, are experienced not separately but in combination, and that we all have different aspects of social identity that coexist with one another. Intersectionality therefore looks at the 'axes of inequality' in combination.[23] It also considers gender and ethnicity as social factors rather than simply demographic ones, viewing them as socially structured, constructed and experienced. So, for example, health differences between men and women arise not just because of biological differences but as a result of the social construction of sex-related roles and relationships (gender). Likewise, ethnic inequalities in health can arise through racism, with ethnic minority groups more likely to experience discrimination personally, institutionally (structural discrimination), and economically.[24] Health inequalities are experienced intersectionally.[25,26]

These inequalities in health result from the unequal distribution across society of the social determinants of health and health-related practices.[27] The social determinants of health are the conditions under which people are born, grow, live, work, and age.[28,29] They are the everyday conditions which influence our access to health-enhancing goods and which limit our exposure to health-damaging risk factors. They include economic resources, as they can determine our ability to afford, or access, good quality services (for example, hospitals, schools, transport infrastructure, and social care), but also allow us to avoid materially harmful circumstances (for example, poor housing, inadequate diet, physical hazards at work, environmental exposures). Besides income, the social determinants of health also include working conditions, housing and neighbourhood factors, labour market activity including unemployment and welfare receipt, and access to certain goods and services such as health and social care. For example, in the US, over 10% of African Americans were uninsured, compared with 6% of non-Hispanic Whites.[30]

These factors can have direct impacts on health (for example, respiratory illnesses are associated with poor-quality damp housing) but can also operate through psychosocial pathways (for example, the chronic stress resulting from insecure housing). Different socioeconomic groups are unequally exposed to these health-damaging or health-enhancing factors, resulting in health inequalities. Another way in which our socioeconomic position in society influences our health is through shaping our health-related practices (often called health behaviours: the ways people spend their time) (for example, exercise) and our forms of consumption that affect health (including diet and tobacco or alcohol use). These socially-shaped health-related practices influence the size and shape of health inequalities; for example, smoking is a social practice which reflects gender roles, social class structures, and income inequalities.[31,32] Most of these health practices are also linked to the 'commercial determinants of health': the companies that manufacture, market and sell unhealthy products, such as tobacco, alcohol and ultra-processed food.[33] Once again, these impacts are unequal, with companies often targeting unhealthy products and services at more marginalised groups. For example, in some US cities there are more fast-food outlets in areas with predominantly Black residents compared to areas with predominantly White residents;[34] in Scotland, alcohol, fast food, tobacco, and gambling outlets have been found to cluster in poorer areas;[35] while global tobacco, alcohol and food companies often exploit gender norms and target racial/ethnic minorities.[36]

Perfect storm: syndemic pandemic[37]

The COVID-19 pandemic is occurring against a backdrop of social and economic inequalities in existing NCDs, as well as inequalities in the social determinants of health. These conditions are creating a horrifying 'perfect storm'. Inequalities in COVID-19 infection and death rates are arising as a result of a syndemic of COVID-19, inequalities in chronic diseases, and the social and commercial determinants of health. The prevalence and severity of the COVID-19 pandemic is magnified because of the preexisting epidemics of chronic disease, which are themselves socially patterned and associated with the social and commercial factors that shape health.

The concept of a syndemic was originally derived from understanding the relationships between HIV/AIDS, substance use, and violence in the US in the 1990s.[38] A syndemic exists when risk factors or co-morbidities are intertwined, interactive and cumulative; that is, when multiple causes of ill health pile upon and reinforce each other in ways that make illness from

COVID-19 more common and more damaging: 'A syndemic is a set of closely intertwined and mutual enhancing health problems that significantly affect the overall health status of a population within the context of a perpetuating configuration of noxious social conditions'.[39] We argue that, for the most disadvantaged communities, COVID-19 is experienced as a syndemic: a co-occurring, synergistic pandemic which interacts with and exacerbates existing chronic health and social conditions.

There are at least four potential pathways that link inequality to higher COVID-19 infection rates, number of cases, case severity and deaths: increased vulnerability, susceptibility, exposure and transmission:[40,41]

- **Increased vulnerability** due to higher burden of preexisting health conditions (such as diabetes and respiratory conditions, heart disease, obesity) that increase the severity and mortality of COVID-19. These comorbidities arise as a result of inequalities in the social determinants of health (for example, working conditions, unemployment, access to essential goods and services, housing and access to healthcare, health-related practices).
- **Increased susceptibility** due to immune systems weakened by long-term exposures to adverse living and environmental conditions. The social determinants of health also work to make people from deprived communities more vulnerable to infection from COVID-19, even when they have no underlying health conditions, as adverse psychosocial circumstances (chronic stress) increase susceptibility, thereby influencing the onset, course and outcome of infectious diseases, including respiratory diseases like COVID-19.
- **Increased exposure** as a result of inequalities in working conditions. Lower-paid workers, particularly in the service sector (for example, food, cleaning or delivery services), were much more likely to be designated as key workers and therefore were still required to go to work during lockdown,

and more likely to be reliant on public transport for doing so. Likewise, people in lower-skilled occupations are less likely to be able to work from home.

- **Increased transmission** – inequalities in housing conditions may also be contributing to inequalities in COVID-19. Deprived neighbourhoods are more likely to contain houses of multiple occupation and smaller houses with a lack of outside space, as well as having higher population densities (particularly in deprived urban areas) and lower access to communal green space. These may have increased COVID-19 transmission rates.

The rest of the book

We submitted this book to the publishers in January 2021, when the pandemic in Europe was in its second wave. Our work is limited to data from 2020. We have used examples from across a variety of countries, though we most often draw on studies from the UK, the US and Canada, partly reflecting our own backgrounds but also because research on inequalities and COVID-19 had been conducted in these countries and was accessible.

The following five chapters examine different aspects of the pandemic and inequality: inequalities in mortality and morbidity; inequalities in the experiences of the lockdown; inequalities in the impacts of the economic crisis; and how these inequalities relate to public policy processes.

Chapter Two, 'Pale rider: pandemic inequalities'

COVID-19 deaths are twice as high in the most deprived neighbourhoods of England and the US than in the most affluent; infection rates are higher in the more deprived regions, such as the northeast of England, and in urban compared to rural areas. There are also significant inequalities by ethnicity and race, with the mortality of minority ethnic groups being considerably higher in many contexts (for example, the death rates for Black Americans in US cities such as Chicago are more than three times as high as for their White counterparts). The average age of death for more marginalised groups is also lower. This chapter will outline these inequalities by drawing on historical and contemporary international evidence of inequalities in influenza pandemics, ranging from the Spanish flu pandemic of 1918 to the H1N1 outbreak of 2009, and current estimates of socioeconomic, racial/ethnic and geographical inequalities in the COVID-19 pandemic. The chapter will also further examine the causes of these inequalities in terms of the syndemic pandemic: the unequal burden of clinical risk factors (such as diabetes, respiratory disease) and the relationship to preexisting inequalities in the social determinants of health.

Chapter Three, 'Collateral damage: inequalities in the lockdown'

This chapter will examine how lockdown experiences were shaped by inequality. While traditional public health surveillance measures of contact tracing and individual quarantine were successfully pursued by some countries (notably by South Korea and Germany), most other countries failed to do so and governments worldwide were eventually forced to implement mass quarantine measures to increase social and physical distancing: lockdowns. These state imposed restrictions – usually requiring governments to take on emergency powers – have been implemented to varying levels of severity, but all have in common a significant increase in social isolation and confinement within the home and immediate neighbourhood for substantial periods (for example, 10–12 weeks). This chapter will examine the unequal social and economic impacts of lockdown experiences (for example, due to job and income loss, overcrowding, urbanity, access to green space, key worker roles), and consider the inequalities arising from the immediate health impacts of these measures (for example, in mental health and gender-based violence).

Chapter Four, 'Pandemic precarity: inequalities in the economic crisis'

This chapter will examine the COVID-19 economic crisis – an economic shock of rare and extreme impact. COVID-19 has had a devastating impact on the world economy: with stock market volatility, oil prices have crashed and there are record levels of unemployment (for example, 5.2 million people filed for unemployment benefit in just one week in the US). It is widely feared that the economic impact will be far greater than the global financial crisis of 2007/8, and that it is likely to be worse in depth than the Great Depression of the 1930s. The economic fallout from the COVID-19 pandemic will have huge consequences for health and health inequalities. This chapter will provide an overview of the unequal impacts of the COVID-19 economic crisis. It will then use evidence from previous recessions – such as the global financial crisis of 2007/8 – to explore the likely unequal health impacts and reflect on the role of social safety nets in preventing them.

Chapter Five, 'Pandemic politics: inequality through public policy'

This chapter argues that the unequal impact of the pandemic was not inevitable. Many politicians have argued that this was a 'black swan' event of extreme rarity, impact and retrospective predictability (black swans come out of nowhere to derail the economy; they are so-called because of an old saying that black swans did not exist, until they were discovered in Western Australia, proving otherwise). The reality is that the pandemic was an entirely predictable 'white swan', whose most devastating effects could have been avoided through better preparation. Indeed, the threat of growing inequities resulting from COVID-19 was more like a 'grey rhino' – a threat that is predictable, not to say obvious – in the light of existing warnings and visible evidence. The chapter reflects on this by comparing country responses, demonstrating that countries with higher rates of social inequality and less generous social security systems had a more unequal pandemic. It will examine variation across and within countries, showing how public policy responses differed and considering how this may have mitigated or exacerbated inequalities in the pandemic and its aftermath.

Chapter Six, 'Conclusion: health and inequality beyond COVID-19'

The book concludes by reflecting on the longer-term implications of the pandemic for social, economic and health inequalities, setting out the type of politics and public policy responses needed to ensure that health inequalities do not increase for future generations and in future pandemics.

TWO

Pale rider: pandemic inequalities

> I looked, and behold, a pale horse; and he who sat on it had the name Death … to kill with sword and with famine and with pestilence.
>
> Book of Revelation 6: 7–8

Introduction

In 1931 Edgar Sydenstricker identified inequalities in the 1918 Spanish flu epidemic, reporting a significantly higher incidence among the working classes.[1] This challenged the widely-held popular, political and scientific consensus of the time that held 'the flu hit the rich and the poor alike'.[2] In the 2020 COVID-19 pandemic, there have been parallel claims made by politicians and the media: that we are 'all in it together' and that the COVID-19 virus 'does not discriminate'.[3] These claims fly in the face of the significant evidence that the pandemic does in fact kill unequally: COVID-19 deaths are twice as high in the most deprived neighbourhoods as in the most affluent; infection rates are higher in more deprived regions, among people with low incomes, and in urban compared to rural areas. There are also even more stark inequalities by ethnicity and race, with the death rates of minority ethnic communities in the UK, Canada and the US being more than twice as high as their majority White counterparts.

This chapter outlines these inequalities, drawing on historical and contemporary international evidence of inequalities in previous respiratory pandemics, ranging from the Spanish flu pandemic of 1918 to the H1N1 outbreak of 2009 and current estimates of social, ethnic and geographical inequalities in the COVID-19 pandemic. It also examines the causes of these inequalities in terms of the unequal burden of risk factors (such as diabetes and respiratory diseases) and the relationship to preexisting inequalities in the social determinants of health, arguing that COVID-19 is a syndemic pandemic. It concludes by reflecting on the longer-term implications of these health inequalities.

An unequal pandemic

In the very first stages of the pandemic (March to June 2020), it quickly became evident, from the experiences of a variety of countries, that there were significant social and ethnic inequalities in COVID-19 infections, symptom severity, hospitalisation and deaths.

Deprivation and COVID-19

The first evidence emerged from data published by the Catalonian government in Spain in April 2020, which suggested that the incident rate of COVID-19 infection was 2.5 times greater in the most deprived areas of Barcelona compared to the least deprived.[4] Similarly, early US analysis from New York City and Illinois – the epicentre of the American pandemic – found clear inequalities between more and less advantaged neighbourhoods in terms of infection levels, with dramatically higher rates among residents of the most disadvantaged areas (367.7 per 100,000 vs. 155.3 per 100,000).[5] In Canada, as early as May 2020, a higher percentage of cases was observed in low-income neighbourhoods. For example, in Toronto, the lowest-income neighbourhoods had significantly higher rates of COVID-19 cases (113 cases per 100,000) and hospitalisations (20 hospitalisations per 100,000), compared to the highest income neighbourhoods (73 cases per 100,000; 9 hospitalisations per 100,000).[6] Similarly, in England, 45% of patients admitted to hospital with COVID-19 were from the most deprived 20% of the population. COVID-19 admissions to critical care were also far greater in the most deprived areas, with over 50% of admissions coming from the 40% most deprived areas.[7,8] A study of primary-care patients in England found that people living in deprived areas were more likely to test positive for COVID-19.[9] Likewise, wide-scale analysis of positive cases by Public Health England (PHE) (from 1 March to 9 May 2020) found that diagnosis rates were highest in the most-deprived quintile (over 300 cases per 100,000), for both men and women – almost double that of the least-deprived quintile (around 200 cases per 100,000).[10] Indeed, the rate in the most-deprived quintile was 1.9 times the rate in the least-deprived quintile among men, and 1.7 times among women. This is particularly concerning in light of growing evidence of 'long COVID', whereby patients have long-term impacts from infection, including neurological and respiratory symptoms as well as fatigue.[11] Lower socioeconomic groups could disproportionately experience these long-term impacts.

These social inequalities in infections, symptom severity, and hospitalisation are also reflected in COVID-19 related deaths. The Illinois and New York City study found a dramatically increased risk of death from COVID-19 among residents of the most disadvantaged areas in the US: COVID-19 death rates were more than double among those living in the most-disadvantaged versus most-advantaged counties (19.3 per 100,000 vs. 9.9 per 100,000; see Table 2.1).[12] Similarly, in Stockholm, Sweden, the highest excess mortality related to

Table 2.1: COVID-19 death rates by county-level poverty, US (March and April 2020)

County % living in poverty		Number of COVID-19 deaths	Population	Death rate per 100,000
Lowest poverty rate	0–4.9	443	4,495,932	9.9
	5–9.9	7,877	71,157,744	11.1
	10–14.9	8,031	108,820,591	7.4
	15–19.9	6,654	101,961,251	6.5
Highest poverty rate	20–100	7,034	36,428,205	19.3

Source: data from Chen and Krieger, 2020.

COVID-19 in March, April and May 2020 occurred in those areas of the city with the lowest income, lowest education, lowest share of Swedish-born people, and the lowest share of employment.[13]

In the early phase of the pandemic (1 March to 31 May 2020) the death rate in the 20% most-deprived English neighbourhoods were 128.3 deaths per 100,000 compared to 58.8 deaths per 100,000 in the least-deprived 20%.[14] Even in the summer of 2020, when the death rates in all areas fell considerably, they were still double in the most-deprived at 3.1 deaths per 100,000 versus 1.4 deaths per 100,000 in the least-deprived neighbourhoods (1 March to 31 July 2020).[15] These inequalities are similar across the different countries of the UK: for example, the COVID-19 death rate among people living in the 20% most-deprived Scottish areas of 86.5 per 100,000 was more than double that of 38.2 in the least-deprived 20% (1 March to 31 May 2020).[16]

There is also evidence of regional inequalities within COVID-19 death rates. In England, mortality rates during the first wave of COVID-19 (March to July 2020) were higher in the northern regions (North East, North West, Yorkshire and Humber) than in the south of England: there were an additional 12.4 COVID-19 deaths per 100,000 people in the northern regions than in the southern ones, and 57.7 more people per 100,000 died in the northern regions than the rest of England from all causes of death.[17]

Although the data in this section so far relate to a small number of high-income settings (notably the US and the UK, both of which have a longstanding research focus on health inequalities and good data availability), there is no reason to assume that the unequal impacts of the pandemic are restricted to these settings. Indeed, emerging evidence from a small number of middle-income countries with high rates of COVID-19 suggests the pattern of both higher incidence and higher mortality in more deprived communities is being repeated. In Brazil, analyses of the Aracaju and São Paulo municipalities suggest that, although more socioeconomically disadvantaged areas initially recorded lower rates of COVID-19, the mortality rates have been higher (increasingly so, over time) and researchers have suggested that lower recorded rates in more disadvantaged areas are partly a reflection of the more limited access to testing resources.[18] Early analyses of metropolitan areas in Chile reaches similar conclusions; while cases were initially higher in more socioeconomically advantaged areas (where the first cases occurred), over time the distribution has shifted to the more vulnerable neighbourhoods.[19] Similarly, analysis of data from the Kolkata megacity region, which has been one of the worst affected areas of India, suggests that COVID-19 hotspots cluster in urban areas of poverty.[20]

Occupational inequalities in COVID-19

In terms of inequalities by occupation, large-scale analysis by the Office of National Statistics (ONS) found that in England

and Wales, COVID-19 death rates in the first wave (March to May 2020) were highest among men employed in:

- elementary occupations (for example, construction workers, security guards, factory workers, and cleaners) with 39.7 deaths per 100,000;
- caring, leisure and other service occupations (for example, nursing assistants, care workers and ambulance drivers) at 39.6 deaths per 100,000;
- process, plant and machine operative occupations at 30.1 deaths per 100,000;
- administrative and secretarial occupations at 26.0 deaths per 100,000;
- sales and customer service occupations at 24.7 deaths per 100,000;
- skilled trades occupations at 23.9 deaths per 100,000.

COVID-19 death rates were lowest among men employed as managers, directors, senior officials and in professional occupations.[21] Similar patterns of occupational inequalities were also evident in the other countries of the UK (for example, in Scotland).[22]

Occupational inequalities in COVID-19 death rates were not as pronounced among women in England and Wales. However, the highest death rates were among women employed in caring, leisure and other service occupations, which had a rate of 15.4 deaths per 100,000 women. Rates were also particularly high among women care workers and home care workers (25.9 deaths per 100,000). Process, plant and machine operatives also had an elevated rate, as did sales and retail assistants (15.7 deaths per 100,000) and national government administrative occupations (23.4 deaths per 100,000). In contrast, COVID-19 death rates were lowest among women employed as managers, directors, senior officials and in professional occupations.[23]

Californian research also noted significant occupational inequalities.[24] Mortality increased by 22% among working-age adults during the first wave of the pandemic (March to June 2020), but this excess mortality was highest in food/agriculture workers (39% increase), transportation/logistics workers (28% increase), and manufacturing workers (23% increase). Occupational impacts were even higher for ethnic minority workers: Latino food/agriculture workers experienced a 59% increase, Black retail workers a 36% increase, and Asian healthcare workers a 40% increase.[25] German research found that COVID-19 hospitalisation rates varied by employment situation, with the long-term unemployed almost twice as likely to be hospitalised as those in employment.[26] In Sweden (which has an advanced welfare state and where equality is regarded as an important policy goal; see Chapter Five), which chose not to lock down to the same extent as its European neighbours or the UK, the inequitable impacts of COVID-19 by occupation still seem similar to the UK; research suggests the highest COVID-19 risks are among taxi and transit drivers, restaurant workers, translators, ambulatory service workers, firefighters, building caretakers, and janitors.[27]

At the time of going to press, there were very few analyses of COVID-19 infection or mortality rates by occupation/employment status in low and middle-income settings. However, concerns about some specifically vulnerable employee populations were being voiced. In India, for example, the sudden government decision to enforce a strict lockdown, in March 2020, left millions of migrant workers in the informal sector with no choice but to return to their rural homes, triggering concerns that this mass migration from urban to rural areas (combined with extreme overcrowding on some trains and buses) was increasing the exposure to COVID-19, not only of these populations but also of their home communities in rural areas.[28]

Racial/ethnic inequalities in COVID-19

COVID-19 inequalities by ethnicity, particularly in the US, are even more stark. Again, evidence emerged quickly of higher rates of infection, symptom severity, hospitalisations and deaths. Surveys conducted in Atlanta and Indiana, during April and May 2020, found that while only around 2% to 3% of all people had the SARS-CoV-2 antibodies, indicating past infection, over 5% of Black and Hispanic participants had the antibodies, indicating that they have been disproportionally affected by the COVID-19 pandemic.[29,30] Research into confirmed cases in Illinois and positive test results in New York City found that the infection rate was more than three times as high during the early stages of the pandemic in communities with a high proportion of ethnic minorities, compared to those with a low proportion (447.0 per 100,000 vs. 127.8 per 100,000).[31] Similarly, in Canada, data shows that neighbourhoods with the highest percentage of people from Black, Asian and minority ethnic (BAME) communities had higher COVID-19 case and hospitalisation rates compared to quintiles with the lowest percentage of each.[32] In Toronto, areas with the highest percentage of recent immigrants also had the highest rate of COVID-19 cases, with 104 per 100,000 people compared to 69 cases per 100,000 people in areas with low levels of recent immigrants.[33] This was reflected in terms of inequalities in hospitalisations: areas with the highest percentage of recent immigrants had the highest rate (18 cases per 100,000 people compared to 8 cases per 100,000 people in areas with the lowest levels of immigration).[34]

These higher rates of illness were also unfortunately reflected in higher death rates. For example, official data from England has found that BAME populations have a much higher death risk than the White British population: compared to White British populations, Black British and Bangladeshi British populations have twice the death risk, with between 10% and 50% greater risk seen across the Indian, Pakistani, Other Asian,

Chinese, Caribbean and Other Black ethnic groups.[35] Similarly, analysis of data from Aotearoa in New Zealand suggests the infection fatality rate for Māori residents is around 50% higher than for non-Māori residents.[36] Even more stark is the data on ethnic inequalities in COVID-19 deaths that is being released by various states and municipalities in the US. For example, in Chicago (period ending 2 July 2020), 75% of COVID-19 deaths were among Black and Latino residents; the COVID-19 death rate for Black Chicagoans is 145 per 100,000 people and 108 per 100,000 for Latino Chicagoans, compared to 56 per 100,000 among White residents.[37,38] Even among children and young people, where symptoms associated with COVID-19 infection are milder and mortality is considerably lower, there were still extreme inequalities, with Hispanic, non-Hispanic Black and non-Hispanic American Indian/Alaskan Native persons accounting for almost 80% of COVID-19 deaths among under-21-year-olds.[39]

This has led some analysts to highlight the underpinning role of systemic and institutional racism (for example, deliberate social policies of residential segregation in the US).[40] In short, historical and institutional racism explain why minority ethnic groups are more likely to live in deprived circumstances in the first place, and why their jobs often lead to greater exposure to COVID-19.[41] This has led Gravlee to also apply the syndemic concept to explain how racism is currently intersecting with the pandemic in the US.[42]

Intersectional inequalities in COVID-19

Of course, people often experience multiple, interacting aspects of inequality at any one time, such as age, gender, occupation, deprivation or race/ethnicity. Each of these 'axes of inequality' influences their health and their experience of the COVID-19 pandemic. Research conducted in Chicago and Cook County, Illinois, demonstrated interactions between race/ethnicity/ age/deprivation.[43] In all racial/ethnic groups and for all ages, mortality was highest in high-poverty neighbourhoods. For younger people (age 0–64 years), White Americans living in high-poverty neighbourhoods died at rates similar to Black Americans living in high-poverty neighbourhoods, but Black Americans and Latino Americans living in low-poverty neighbourhoods died at almost three times the rate of White Americans in similar neighbourhoods. For older people (age 65 years +) there was clear 'White advantage' in COVID-19 mortality across all income groups. Even White Americans living in the highest-poverty neighbourhoods were less likely to die of COVID-19 than the wealthiest Black/Latino Americans. This suggests that racial/ethnic inequalities in COVID-19 mortality interact with socioeconomic and institutional factors (for example, structural racism).[44]

The ghost of pandemics past

These inequalities in the 2020 COVID-19 pandemic reflect longstanding patterns of social inequalities in health, evident across multiple illnesses and causes of death and even evident in previous pandemics. There were significant inequalities in the 2009 H1N1 influenza pandemic, for example, as the mortality rate in the most deprived quintile of England's population was three times higher than in the least deprived.[45] This is shown in Table 2.2. It was also higher in urban compared to rural areas.[46] Similarly, in Canada, hospitalisation rates for H1N1 were associated with lower educational attainment and living in a high deprivation neighbourhood.[47] In the US, people with financial problems (for example, financial barriers to healthcare access) were more likely to report H1N1 symptoms.[48] We also see inequalities every year in mortality, morbidity and symptom severity with cyclical winter flu among both adults and children.[49,50]

However, it was over a hundred years ago, in 1918, that the world last experienced a pandemic on the scale of COVID-19. The so-called Spanish flu pandemic (named because the

Table 2.2: Death rates due to pandemic (H1N1) 2009 influenza in England (1 June 2009–18 April 2010) by quintile of neighbourhood deprivation

Quintile of deprivation		Population (thousands)	Deaths	Death rate (per million people)
Least deprived	5	10,289	42	3.9
	4	10,289	56	5.3
	3	10,289	53	5.1
	2	10,289	80	7.8
Most deprived	1	10,289	118	12.0

Source: data from Rutter et al, 2012.

first newspaper reports of the pandemic emerged in Spain, though it is now thought to have originated within the Allied armies) swept across the globe in three waves, infecting 500 million people, a third of the world's population, leading to an estimated 50–100 million deaths, with rates particularly high in war-ravaged Europe.[51] Death was particularly high in young children, those aged between 20 and 40 years (a unique feature of this pandemic), as well as older people.[52] And, as Edgar Sydenstricker asserted in 1931, there were significant inequalities, with historical research now demonstrating that there were clear social and geographical inequalities in the impact of the Spanish flu. Infection and death rates were substantially higher in less affluent neighbourhoods; among the working classes; and in urban areas. In Norway, death rates were highest in the working-class districts of Oslo;[53] in the US they were highest among the unemployed and the urban poor;[54] in Australia death levels were lower among professional and commercial groups and higher in lower status occupations, such as labourers;[55] and in Sweden deaths were higher in the lowest occupational classes.[56] These social inequalities were particularly great among men.[57] There were also urban–rural differences noted, whereby, for example, in England and Wales, mortality was 30% to 40% higher in urban areas.[58] There is also some evidence from the US that the pandemic had long-term impacts on inequalities in child health and development.[59] However, this was not the case everywhere: countries with smaller preexisting social and economic inequalities, such as New Zealand, did not experience any socioeconomic inequalities in mortality during the 1918 pandemic.[60,61]

England and Wales provide an interesting and well-documented case study of inequalities in the Spanish flu, as the Registrar General Sir Bernard Mallet (the top government official for medical statistics) published a large report in 1920, providing crude death rates by locality across England and Wales alongside some analysis of regional and social inequalities.[62] Figure 2.1 maps the final death rates from all three waves of the Spanish flu pandemic in England. It shows strong geographical inequalities across England, with the northern districts and counties having a much higher total death rate than the southern ones. Indeed, Table 2.3 shows that the places with the highest death rates were all located in the North or the Midlands (and Wales), while the areas with the lowest death rates were all located in the South. At the extremes, the geographical inequalities were such that the death rate recorded in Hebburn near Newcastle in the northeast of England (1194 per 100,000) was six times that of the lowest in Sutton in Surrey in the southeast (188 per 100,000). These regional inequalities were noted at the time, with the Registrar General concluding that the North and the Midlands experienced a higher level of death. He commented that 'the northern parts of the country suffered decidedly more, on the whole, than the southern'.[63] Indeed, data from his 1920 report shows that the North (540 per 100,000 people) and the Midlands (490 per 100,000 people) suffered the highest death rates and the South (440 per 100,000 people) the least. London was the same as the national average at 490 per 100,000 people.

Figure 2.1: Map of local mortality rates from 1918 Spanish Flu pandemic per 100,000 population (categorised into quintiles), England and Wales

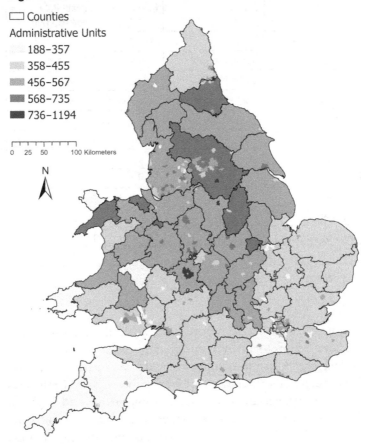

☐ Counties
Administrative Units
188–357
358–455
456–567
568–735
736–1194

0   25   50   100 Kilometers

N

Source: reproduced under creative commons licence from Bambra et al, 2020c.

Recent analysis by the historical geographer Niall Johnson found that northern cities had higher rates of death in all three waves of the Spanish flu pandemic.[64] Together, this suggests that urban areas, coastal areas, and areas well-served by mass

Table 2.3: English towns with highest and lowest death rates from the 1918 Spanish Flu

Town	County	Region	Death Rate per 100,000
Highest Rates			
Hebburn	Durham	North	1,194
Jarrow	Durham	North	877
Kidderminster	Worcestershire	Midlands	849
Barnsley	Yorkshire	North	835
Wallsend	Northumberland	North	828
Lowest Rates			
Hereford	Herefordshire	South	277
Sutton	Surrey	South	188
Woking	Surrey	South	225
Winchester	Hampshire	South	250
Taunton	Somerset	South	272

Source: Johnson, 2001.

communication and transport links, suffered higher infection and death rates than rural, inland and isolated areas.[65]

Poverty, deprivation, sanitation and overcrowding may also have been important factors behind the higher death rates in the northern areas. However, looking beyond regional inequalities, that there were wider social inequalities in the impact of the Spanish flu pandemic was contested at the time, and has been a source of controversy among historians ever since.[66] The Registrar General, certain local medical officers and commentators claimed at the time that it was 'a matter of common knowledge that the pandemic... affected all classes of the population irrespective of their social and economic status, or even of their personal vigour and physique'.[67] In contrast, the County Medical Officer and School Medical Officer for the County of London, William Hamer, argued that 'total mortality... was conditioned by the social class of the population'.[68] When examining data from across the different boroughs of London, Niall Johnson found that – just like with COVID-19 and deprivation – there was a clear association between influenza mortality and household wealth (percentage of houses with domestic servants) and preexisting health indicators (infant mortality rates). The most affluent London borough, then and now: Kensington, had the lowest death rate from the Spanish flu (340 per 100,000 people), while St Pancras, the poorest borough – and still one of the poorest – had the highest (620 per 100,000 people).[69] Further analysis for the whole of England and Wales also found relationships between influenza deaths and pre-pandemic mortality rates (which are themselves closely correlated with poverty, deprivation, sanitation and overcrowding).[70] Interestingly, this analysis also found a relationship with deprivation levels today.

So, social inequality mattered in 1918: more affluent people, areas and regions had a better Spanish flu pandemic. They may have been better able to avoid the disease than poorer communities living in overcrowded homes and working in factories; more affluent sections of the population would also have had better healthcare resources, better preexisting health status (for example, from better diets and nutritional intake), and better housing conditions. All of which increased their survival chances, and, as the next section outlines, these aspects of inequality are also important over a century later when examining the shape of the COVID-19 pandemic.

The syndemic of COVID-19 and inequality[71]

As in 1918, the COVID-19 pandemic is occurring against a backdrop of social and economic inequalities in existing NCDs, as well as inequalities in the social determinants of health. Inequalities in COVID-19 infection and death rates are therefore arising as a result of a syndemic of COVID-19, inequalities in chronic diseases, and the social determinants of health. The prevalence and severity of the COVID-19 pandemic is magnified because of the preexisting epidemics of chronic disease, which are themselves socially patterned and associated with the social determinants of health. The concept of a syndemic was originally derived from understanding the relationships between HIV/AIDS, substance use, and violence in the US in the 1990s.[72] A syndemic exists when risk factors or comorbidities are intertwined, interactive and cumulative, adversely exacerbating the disease burden and additively increasing its negative effects: 'A syndemic is a set of closely intertwined and mutual enhancing health problems that significantly affect the overall health status of a population within the context of a perpetuating configuration of noxious social conditions'.[73] We argue that for the most disadvantaged communities, COVID-19 is experienced as a syndemic: a co-occurring, synergistic pandemic which interacts with and exacerbates their existing chronic health and social conditions (Figure 2.2).

Minority ethnic groups, people living in areas of higher social deprivation, those in poverty, and other marginalised groups (such as homeless people, prisoners, and street-based sex workers) generally have a greater number of coexisting chronic health conditions which are more severe, and they experience them at a younger age. Research has shown that chronic conditions (such as hypertension, diabetes, asthma, COPD, heart, liver, and renal disease, cancer, cardiovascular disease, obesity and smoking) increase the likelihood of complications and deaths due to COVID-19. For example, people with diabetes are three times more likely to experience severe symptoms or death from COVID-19,[74] smokers are one-and-a-half times more likely to experience severe symptoms,[75] and the odds of developing severe COVID-19 are up to seven times higher in obese patients.[76] People living in more socially disadvantaged neighbourhoods, and minority ethnic groups, have higher rates of almost all of these known underlying

Figure 2.2: The syndemic of COVID-19, non-communicable diseases (NCDs) and the social determinants of health

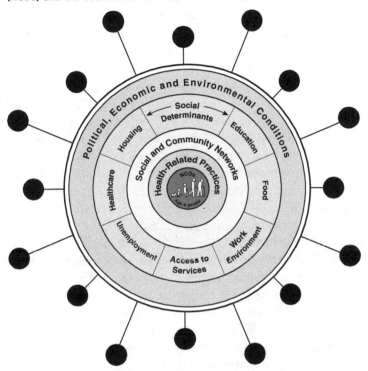

Source: reproduced from Bambra et al, 2020a, with permission of BMJ publishing group.

clinical risk factors that increase the severity of and death from COVID-19.[77] Similarly, the Gypsy/Roma community – one of the most marginalised minority groups in Europe – has a smoking rate that is two to three times the European average, increased rates of respiratory diseases (such as COPD), and other COVID-19 risk factors.[78]

These inequalities in chronic conditions arise as a result of inequalities in exposure to the social determinants of health: the conditions in which people 'live, work, grow and age' including working conditions, unemployment, access to essential goods and services (for example, water, sanitation and food), housing, and access to healthcare.[79,80] By way of example, there are considerable occupational inequalities in exposure to adverse working conditions (for example, ergonomic hazards, repetitive work, long hours, shift work, low wages, job insecurity); they are concentrated in lower-skill jobs. These working conditions are associated with increased risks of respiratory diseases, certain cancers, musculoskeletal disease, hypertension, stress and anxiety.[81] In addition to these long-term exposures, inequalities in working conditions may well be impacting on the unequal distribution of the COVID-19 disease burden. For example, lower-paid workers, where BAME groups are disproportionately represented, particularly in the service sector (for example, food, cleaning or delivery services), are less likely to be able to work from home and much more likely to be designated as key workers, and thereby still required to go into work even during lockdowns. They are also much more likely to be reliant on public transport. Insecure work, and lack of sick pay from employers and the state, also reduce the ability for these communities to self-isolate when symptomatic. All of this increases their exposure to the virus.

Similarly, access to healthcare is lower in disadvantaged and marginalised communities, even in universal healthcare systems.[82] In England, the number of patients per general practitioner is 15% higher in the most-deprived areas than in the least-deprived.[83] Medical care is even more unequally distributed in countries such as the US where around 33 million Americans, from the most disadvantaged and marginalised groups, have insufficient or no healthcare insurance.[84] This reduced access to healthcare, before and during the outbreak, contributes to inequalities in chronic disease and is also likely to lead to worse outcomes from COVID-19 in the more disadvantaged areas and marginalised communities. Further, as a result of health services having to focus on combating the pandemic, there has also been a significant reduction in healthcare access for people with existing chronic conditions, such as cancer or cardiovascular disease. Similarly, access to preventative care has also been restricted as a result of healthcare system pressures and the need for social distancing. This is also likely to have a disproportionate impact on low-income and ethnic- minority populations with higher rates of NCDs.

Housing is also an important factor in driving health inequalities.[85] For example, exposure to poor quality housing is associated with certain health outcomes; for instance, damp housing can lead to respiratory diseases such as asthma, while overcrowding can result in higher infection rates and increased risk of injury from household accidents. Overcrowding and less spacious housing is associated with higher CRP (C-Reactive Protein) levels, a biomarker of inflammation and stress.[86] Housing also impacts on health inequalities materially through costs (for example, as a result of high rents), and psychosocially through insecurity (for example, short-term leases). Lower social groups have a higher exposure to poor-quality or unaffordable, insecure housing, and therefore have a higher rate of the negative health consequences.[87] These inequalities in housing conditions may also be contributing to inequalities in COVID-19. For example, deprived neighbourhoods are more likely to contain houses of multiple occupation, smaller houses with a lack of outside space, higher population densities (particularly in deprived urban areas), and less access to communal green space.[88] These will likely increase COVID-19 transmission rates, as was the case with H1N1 where strong associations were found with urbanity.[89]

The social determinants of health also work to make people from marginalised communities more vulnerable to infection from COVID-19, even when they have no underlying health conditions. Decades of research into the psychosocial determinants of health have found that the chronic stress of material and psychological deprivation is associated with immunosuppression.[90] Psychosocial feelings of subordination or inferiority, as a result of occupying a low position on the social hierarchy, stimulate physiological stress responses (for example, raised cortisol levels) which, when prolonged (chronic), can have long-term adverse consequences for physical and mental health.[91] By way of example, studies have found consistent associations between low job status (for example, low control and high demands), stress-related morbidity, and various chronic conditions including coronary heart disease, hypertension, obesity, musculoskeletal conditions, and psychological ill health.[92] Likewise, there is increasing evidence that living in disadvantaged environments may produce a sense of powerlessness and collective threat among residents, leading to chronic stressors that, in time, damage health.[93] Studies have also confirmed that adverse psychosocial circumstances increase susceptibility, influencing the onset, course and outcome of infectious diseases, including respiratory diseases like COVID-19.[94]

Thus, at least four potential pathways link social inequality to higher COVID-19 infection rates, number of cases, case severity and deaths: increased vulnerability, susceptibility, exposure and transmission (see Chapter One). These consequences of socioeconomic inequality also intersect with ethnicity, as ethnic minorities are much more likely to be socioeconomically deprived and/or to live in more deprived neighbourhoods, as well as to be disproportionally disadvantaged by compounding determinants.[95] There are also intersections with age and gender with, for example, higher rates of death among older age groups and men.[96]

Conclusion

This chapter has summarised the emerging evidence of socioeconomic, geographical and racial/ethnic inequalities in COVID-19 cases, symptom severity and deaths. People living in more deprived neighbourhoods, in lower-paid occupations, and from racial/ethnic minorities, are experiencing worse COVID-19 outcomes with death rates at least twice as high as more privileged groups and places. The chapter has also shown the lessons from history, whereby today we are replicating the patterns of inequality from previous pandemics. Both then and now, these inequalities have emerged through the syndemic nature of COVID-19, as it interacts with and exacerbates existing social inequalities in chronic disease and the social determinants of health. COVID-19 has laid bare our longstanding social, economic, political and health inequalities. In the next chapters, we examine the unequal impacts of the effects of the emergency measures (social distancing and lockdown) implemented in response to COVID-19. Chapter Three examines the unequal experiences of lockdown and in the 'parallel pandemics' of mental health and loneliness. Chapter Four examines the likely impact on health inequalities of the COVID-19 global economic slump.

THREE

Collateral damage: inequalities in the lockdown

When we try to pick out anything by itself, we find it hitched to everything else in the Universe.

John Muir, 1911

Introduction

This chapter explores the 'collateral damage' caused by COVID-19 and subsequent policy responses designed to contain the spread of the virus. While Chapters One, Two and Four focus on some of the direct health and economic consequences of the pandemic, this chapter brings together evidence concerning the inequalities in the multitude of less direct impacts of lockdown policies, highlighting the complex interconnections between the pandemic and our lives: the syndemic pandemic. For the most part, these indirect impacts are, like the health and economic impacts, deeply concerning and unequally spread; those who are less well-off are also often less well protected and so bear the brunt of the 'collateral damage'. However, as we will see in Chapter Six, there are also some glimmers of hope when it comes to considering the indirect impacts of the pandemic, especially when we consider potential coalitions for progressive change.

The chapter is organised around Figure 2.2, so it starts by considering the impacts that are most obviously related to health because they are most proximal (for example, the impacts on NCDs and other health conditions) and then moves out, through the various layers of the rainbow. It closes by considering the uncertainties around how the pandemic might reshape the macro-level political, economic and social conditions in which we live and work (a theme which is picked up again in Chapters Five and Six). Since the evidence on collateral damage is new and emergent, the geopolitical focus of the chapter is diverse, drawing in examples in ways that reflect this growing evidence base, though the UK (where a wealth of relevant research has already been published) features throughout.

It is necessary, therefore, to keep in mind the variations in policy responses across different contexts. While some countries (such as the UK) had repeated lockdowns in which people were asked to stay at home and in which schools and nurseries were closed (initially and subsequently en masse but with more sporadic closures in response to outbreaks in between), other countries (such as Sweden) took a more laissez-faire approach, merely restricting large public gatherings but keeping schools and childcare open. Additionally, a small number of countries (notably New Zealand) locked down early and closed their borders, enabling them to emerge and operate as effectively 'COVID-free', albeit while continuing to maintain strict border controls. These variations, aspects of which are described in Chapter Five as well, have necessarily shaped patterns and experiences of the kinds of collateral damage – and inequalities - that we are now witnessing. This chapter focuses on experiences in countries that have employed lengthy lockdown periods.

Collateral health and wellbeing impacts

The pandemic unfolded in a context of widespread chronic illness. Despite the existence of a Sustainable Development Goal (SDG) to reduce premature mortality (deaths before age 75 years) from NCDs, such as cancer, diabetes and cardiovascular disease, by a third by 2030, and some evidence of overall reductions between 1990 and 2017, progress has been highly uneven.[1] A 2020 *Lancet Global Health* analysis reported that only a small number of countries (mainly in the West Pacific and Europe, almost all high-income settings) were on track to meet this SDG target, while 2017 data indicated 'high premature avertable mortality from NCDs was clustered in low-income and middle-income countries'.[2] Moreover, as Chapter Two of this book highlights, the progress that high-income countries have made in reducing premature mortality from NCDs masks substantial within-country inequalities. In the UK, for example, these inequalities were already so great (pre-pandemic) that, since the early 2010s, previously improving life expectancy and all-cause mortality had already begun to stall, with the most disadvantaged populations experiencing increased mortality, leading to increases in both absolute and relative inequalities.[3] Since many chronic health conditions are risk factors for COVID-19 morbidity and mortality, the likelihood of experiencing major health problems or death from COVID-19 were already uneven.[4]

On top of this, in some countries, health services were unable to cope with simultaneously tackling multiple cases of COVID-19 while also providing care and interventions for existing chronic health conditions. Evidence from England, for example, shows that many previously planned health interventions were postponed as hospitals came under pressure to prioritise treating patients with COVID-19.[5] In other settings, where healthcare was not free at the point of delivery, large sections of the population were already struggling to afford access to healthcare.[6,7] At the same time, evidence from multiple countries suggests that far fewer people than normal are seeking healthcare to explore non-COVID-19 health concerns during the pandemic (for example, symptoms that may be the early signs of cancer or heart disease).[8,9,10,11] A General Practitioner in England summed up her concerns in April 2020, during the first UK lockdown:

> The worry of most GPs at the moment isn't COVID-19, as we are well set up now ... Our worry is that we are not seeing the breast lumps, postnatal depression, pelvic pain, abnormal bleeding, mini-strokes, rectal bleeding, neck lumps, swallowing difficulties, suspicious weight loss, moles that are changing shape, palpitations, chest pain suspicious for angina, abdominal pain suspicious for appendicitis and more. They must be still happening but people are staying at home, 'not wanting to bother us'. (Jennifer Graham, a GP in northern England, 2020)[12]

Since the burden of chronic illness largely follows the social gradient of health (see Chapter One), the impacts of these wider health challenges will inevitably be unequal.[13,14,15] They are also likely to cast a long shadow over health experiences going forward, as healthcare systems struggle to catch up with the growing backlogs of preventative (for example, screening), routine and non-emergency care, much of which relates to NCDs.[16]

This unequal health burden also extends to mental health, across a wide variety of settings. For example, two separate longitudinal studies undertaken in the UK have identified worsening mental health since the outbreak of the COVID-19 pandemic, and highlight inequalities within these findings.[17,18] Both studies found that the mental health of women and young people was particularly affected by the pandemic; one study also identified those with pre-school aged children were more affected,[19] while the other found that people from more socially disadvantaged backgrounds and those with preexisting mental health problems were particularly affected.[20] An online survey conducted in Spain in April and May 2020 also identified worsening mental health in the context of COVID-19 and Spain's first lockdown, and found younger participants (18–35 years), women, and those who perceived their housing to be inadequate were all more affected.[21] Similarly, a survey conducted in China in January and February 2020 identified rising levels of mental distress in the context of COVID-19 and the initial lockdown and found younger participants (18–30 years), women, and migrant workers were most impacted.[22] The findings of these studies seem remarkably consistent considering the diversity of the settings; they all suggest that COVID-19 and the associated lockdown experiences have had a negative impact on mental health and that this impact has been unequal, with women and younger adults faring less well. In all three countries (China, Spain and the UK), there is also evidence that those in less well-off income groups have been hardest hit by the mental health fallout of the pandemic.[23,24,25]

The reasons for this are likely multiple, but make sense in the context of the unequal impacts of the virus. As Chapters One and Two illustrate, socially disadvantaged groups have been more exposed to the virus and have experienced greater rates of mortality – and this means that people in these groups are more likely to be experiencing bereavement and grief, both of which are known to impact on mental health,[26] especially where the loss of a loved one is unexpected.[27] It is also likely that many people in these groups are aware (as a result of widespread media coverage) that they face relatively greater risks, which itself may fuel fear and distress. The 'collateral damage' described in the rest of this chapter, including social, environmental and financial impacts, also helps to explain this inequality. Interestingly, the Chinese survey found that levels of distress seemed lower in parts of China perceived to have a strong public health system, even if rates of COVID-19 were relatively high (for example, Shanghai),[28] which highlights the protective role that strong social policies can provide (as discussed further in Chapter Five).

There is also emerging evidence of ethnic inequalities in the mental health impacts of COVID-19. In the Canadian province of Quebec, for example, an online survey conducted in June 2020 found that the mental health impact of the pandemic varied significantly by socioeconomic status and ethnocultural group, with those on lower incomes and those who identified as belonging to Arab ethnocultural groups reporting higher psychological distress.[29] The same study found that exposure to the virus, COVID-19-related discrimination, and stigma were all associated with poorer mental health, and that these factors were all more prevalent in minority ethnic groups.[30] In the UK, longitudinal survey data suggest that increases in mental distress during the pandemic also vary by ethnicity, with Black, Asian, and minority ethnic men experiencing higher average increases in mental distress than White British men, meaning the gender gap in mental health increases only appears to apply to White British individuals.[31] Perhaps unsurprisingly, given that discrimination, stigma and racism are evident in many contexts, concerns have also been raised about the likelihood of ethnic inequalities in COVID-19-related mental health experiences elsewhere, including in Australia, India, and the US.[32,33,34]

A qualitative study carried out in northern India illustrates how awareness of ethnic differences can, in the context of the heightened risks presented by COVID-19, rapidly translate into experiences of othering, prejudice and stigma for minority groups:

> People from the Muslim community are all not following the rules ... and there is a change in our relations since COVID ... Earlier the women in the neighbourhood used to say 'tum meri dharam ki behen ho' (that you are my sister in faith) but now they are ready to run bulldozers over

our homes. They threaten us over everything, and they are full of hatred. (Female participant, 41 years old, 2020)[35]

This extract powerfully illustrates that, regardless of the accuracy of such perceptions, where particular ethnic groups are perceived as more at risk of carrying COVID-19 this can cause heightened racism and prejudice, which are likely to further exacerbate inequalities in mental health. Similarly, research in the US found, in the context of media and policy framings of COVID-19 as the 'Chinese flu' and the 'Wuhan virus', anti-Asian attitudes were activated.[36]

So far, the collateral health and wellbeing impacts of COVID-19 tell a depressingly familiar tale: largely negative health impacts tend to affect most strongly those who are already at greater risk of ill health. The evidence relating to one set of key risk factors for ill health: the consumption of unhealthy commodities, is, however, a little more uneven. While evidence from several countries suggests lockdown experiences have led to widespread weight gain,[37,38,39] the impact on smoking and alcohol consumption is more mixed, with variations by product and context. For example, evidence from the UK suggests that people reduced rates of smoking during the pandemic;[40] this is in a context in which tobacco control measures are particularly strong.[41] In contrast, evidence suggests that smoking increased during the lockdown in Poland,[42] a context with fewer tobacco control policies.[43] In South Africa, where the government decided to ban the sale of tobacco and alcohol products (as 'non-essential' items),[44] which might have been expected to reduce both smoking and alcohol consumption, emerging evidence (which looked at the numbers of cigarette butts in urban street litter) suggests cigarette consumption did not decline, at least not significantly.[45] More positively, there are early indications that the ban on alcohol reduced alcohol consumption and associated alcohol-related trauma (a welcome development given the strong association between alcohol consumption and violence in South Africa).[46] These experiences may offer lessons for policymakers with a view to improving health and wellbeing beyond the pandemic.[47] In Europe, survey data suggest that alcohol consumption has declined since the outbreak of COVID-19, even in countries that did not ban or restrict alcohol sales.[48] However, this welcome public health news does not appear to have benefited all equally; respondents with high incomes reported more pronounced declines in alcohol consumption than those with low incomes.[49] The UK also appears to be a notable exception, with evidence suggesting there may have been an increase in alcohol consumption in the context of the pandemic.[50,51]

Collateral social and community impacts

A key aspect of the pandemic lockdown experience that helps explain the greater mental health impact on women seems to be the greater levels of caring-related work women have been undertaking. This is partly because caring work, more of which was already undertaken by women around the world prior to the pandemic, has increased as a result of COVID-19 and the associated lockdowns.[52] In April 2020, the UN released a report which highlighted the increase in unpaid care work and the unequal impact on women.[53] This stems from the combined effects of the closures of schools and nurseries (substantially increasing childcare demands) and the increase in the need to care for sick, older and disabled relatives (because they had become ill or because they could no longer access their usual carers, at a time when health and care services have been under unprecedented pressure). Reflecting this, data from an online survey conducted in Germany in the first few weeks of their lockdown (27 March to 26 April 2020) found that women tended to worry more than men about pressures and challenges relating to childcare.[54] A virtual ethnography undertaken in Italy (March to May 2020) found that the lockdown had also exacerbated gender inequality there, heightening unequal domestic arrangements around parenting.[55] For mothers who were also trying to work, this resulted in stress, guilt and a lack of sleep, while some of those who found themselves undertaking domestic work full-time during the lockdown described the relentless nature as crushing:

> I feel very guilty, so I try to get organised: on the round table, we do puzzles, constructions, [and] drawings together. Sometimes I turn on the PC and work while he plays, we don't interact much. There is silence, so I put on some music. It's all horrendous! Perhaps you are in a call with your boss and your son needs to go pee, and you can't understand either one or the other.

> The grievousness of the housework is crushing! For instance, I wash the floors, and then the girl literally pees on it. I make the beds, and a second later they already suck … it's frustrating, and I think 'thank goodness that I don't do this all my life'. (Two separate female participants in an Italian virtual ethnography, 2020)[56]

More disturbingly, evidence is beginning to emerge that charts a rise in violence against women and children during the lockdowns.[57] This trend appears to be international, with reports of increased domestic violence coming from multiple countries, including Australia, China, EU member states, India, Pakistan, the US and the UK.[58,59,60,61,62,63,64] In the UK, a report by Women's Aid, based on a suite of new research, found that over 60% of women surveyed who were living with their abuser reported experiencing an increase in violence and abuse during the lockdown, with one reporting she felt the situation turned her into a 'sitting duck'.[65] Half of the mothers currently experiencing abuse said their children had witnessed more abuse, and over a third said their abuser had increased the abusive behaviour directed towards their children.[66] The indirect impacts of the pandemic on these women and children are multiple: for those living with an abuser, abuse increased substantially during lockdown; some women reported the pandemic being employed as part of the abuse (for example, partners exposing themselves and children to unnecessary danger, refusing to follow hygiene rules, or exerting greater control over food, finances and medicine); for others, simply being less able to leave home and requirements to wear masks brought back memories of past abuse.[67] At the same time, available support declined, with key organisations experiencing a combination of funding crises and a lack of staff (due to illness, shielding, self-isolation, and so on), and government rules limiting socialisation restricting support from agencies, friends and families: 'when he had been abusive no-one would come and help due to the COVID-19. Even when the police said it's ok for someone to come to sit with me no-one would come' (Female abuse survivor, UK).[68]

This clearly impacts on women's physical and mental health; one of the surveys conducted as part of the UK Women's Aid research found over half of the women experiencing abuse during the pandemic reported that their mental health had worsened.[69] Synthesis of available international research has found that lower parental education (an indicator of socioeconomic status) is strongly associated with increased risk of women experiencing intimate partner violence. This means that the impacts of the pandemic and lockdown on violence are, like so many other impacts, likely to be greater for women who are less well-off.[70]

Similar concerns are being raised in regard to rising levels of neglect and abuse of children, particularly in light of school closures and reduced health and social services (teachers, social workers and healthcare practitioners often play a vital role in raising the alarm about children who are experiencing neglect and/or abuse).[71,72] In France, for example, there has been a reduction in official orders to protect children from abuse, but this has occurred alongside a 90% increase in calls to the national child abuse helpline.[73] Similarly, in the US, emergency department visits relating to child abuse and neglect decreased during the pandemic, but the proportion of visits requiring hospitalisation increased (compared to 2019).[74] These kinds of evidence fuel fears that a hidden epidemic of child abuse is occurring in the shadow of COVID-19 – an epidemic that is likely to map onto the wider social inequalities that the pandemic is revealing. Research reporting the voices of frontline workers in the US reported one social worker saying, 'We're not just seeing cracks, we're seeing massive fissures'.[75]

More broadly, there are widespread concerns about the impacts of school closures on children's wellbeing and longer-term educational attainment, with evidence suggesting that the long-term consequences are likely to be significantly greater for children who are already socially disadvantaged. Predicting these impacts is difficult because the current circumstances are so unusual, but researchers in the US used previous findings regarding the effects of other kinds of school closures (for example, as a result of summer holiday periods, weather-related closures and pupil absenteeism) on educational attainment, to try to project the impacts of the initial COVID-19 related school closures.[76] This research suggests that students returning to school in the US in autumn 2020 were, on average, likely to return with only 63–68% of the learning gains in reading and 37–50% of the learning gains in maths relative to a typical school year. However, the projections suggested these averages were likely to mask substantial variations, with the top third of students potentially making gains in reading. Similarly, a rapid review of available evidence which sought to project the likely impact of school closures on inequalities in educational attainment in England found that school closures were likely to widen the attainment gap between disadvantaged children and their peers by over 35%, reversing progress made to narrow the gap since 2011.[77] Likewise, a report working to project the likely consequences for 17 Latin American countries warns that high school completion rates of children with low-educated parents could fall by 20%, 'reversing decades of progress made by the region in terms of educational upward mobility'.[78]

Research to assess the actual impacts on educational attainment is still emerging. However, analysis of longitudinal survey data in the UK revealed that in April 2020, one month after the start of the first lockdown, most children had lost out on education; there were, as expected, substantial inequalities, which meant that children from the most disadvantaged families lost out more than those from the most advantaged.[79] Qualitative research with teachers, undertaken in England, exploring the impacts of the first lockdown, highlight some of the structural challenges that explain these variations in educational outcomes: these included access to hardware and internet services required for online learning, but also basic necessities and wellbeing.[80] Indeed, the researchers identified very high levels of anxiety about disadvantaged pupils, with teachers describing 'feeling powerless to help pupils they are used to looking out for and worried about those whom they may not even have realised were at risk before now'.[81] This research also notes that it is not necessarily easy for basic assessments to pick up the barriers that children are experiencing – for example, one teacher reflected:

> if somebody in authority asked them the question, 'do you have internet access?' they, of course, they would say yes. But in reality what they have is a phone, that's Mum's phone that she can get the internet on ... And Mum is terrified of wasting the data because she's got no money to buy some more. (Teacher, England, 2020)[82]

The space available within the home environment poses additional challenges for children trying to learn from home, adults trying to work at home, and everyone trying to maintain their mental health, exercise and, where necessary, socially distance. Restrictions requiring people to spend far more time at home and to remain socially distant from others are shining a light on the extent of inequalities in housing across diverse settings. In South Africa, for example, a significant proportion of households live in shacks, colloquially named 'bungalows' or 'hokkies', which share boundaries and often incorporate zinc and corrugated iron as well as brick. As De Groot and Lemanski write: 'Not only are neighbouring structures too close to satisfy social distancing requirements, but residents risk exposure to inhumane temperatures if they remain indoors (as non-brick materials magnify outdoor temperatures)'.[83]

Although the extent of poor housing and overcrowding is generally greater in low and middle-income settings, high-income settings are far from immune. In the UK, housing in some urban areas (notably London) has become so expensive that overcrowding and multi-generational households are common.[84] These inequalities have direct and indirect impacts on health and wellbeing in the context of COVID-19. For example, a report by the New Policy Institute think tank, which analysed data on confirmed cases of COVID-19 per head of population across 149 English local authorities, found that the proportion of over-70s who share a household with people of working age was a significant factor in explaining local authority variation in COVID-19 cases.[85] Similarly, analysis of US counties found that, with each 5% increase in the percentage of households with poor housing conditions in the county, there was a 50% higher risk of COVID-19 incidence.[86] Housing quality also impacts people's mental health and wellbeing and their ability to exercise (especially while shielding or self-isolating).[87]

Relatedly, multiple studies have highlighted increased public use of urban greenspaces since the start of pandemic restrictions.[88,89] A survey undertaken in Tokyo (another international city in which the high cost of property drives overcrowding) during the pandemic found that the frequency of greenspace use and the existence of green window views from within the home was associated with increased levels of self-esteem, life satisfaction, and subjective happiness and decreased levels of depression, anxiety, and loneliness.[90] However, concerns have been raised about the possibility of COVID-19 transmission in greenspaces that are particularly well used. A study of greenspace use in England and Wales, for example, found that areas in which more of the housing is made up of flats (which are generally cheaper than houses) tend to be closer to parks, but that people living in these areas often end up visiting parks that can become overcrowded, potentially increasing transmission of COVID-19.[91]

Since both housing and greenspace are unequally distributed, the impacts of the pandemic relating to housing and neighbourhood inevitably fall unequally. In many contexts, there is a link between low incomes, poor housing and lack of access to greenspace; in some countries, historical policies and structural racism mean that poor-quality housing and limited access to greenspace are also more common issues for particular ethnic groups. For example, in Australia, poor-quality housing is particularly concentrated in Aboriginal and Torres Strait Islander populations while, in the US, Black American and Latino communities are more likely to live in urban areas and therefore have lower access to greenspace.[92,93]

Another widely acknowledged consequence of lockdown experiences at the social and community level has been the reduction in social contact, which has stimulated a wealth of concerns about loneliness and isolation: risk factors for worsening mental health. Particular concerns have also been raised, in several settings, about older people and those living alone.[94,95] Part of the concern around older people stems from the 'digital divide', with older generations being less likely to have the skills or resources to maintain social connections virtually.[96] However, a US study suggests that these groups may be relatively resilient to the social isolation caused by lockdown measures.[97] Using survey data, researchers examined changes in loneliness in response to the social restriction measures in a nationwide sample of US adults.[97] Surprisingly, they found no significant changes in loneliness and, although older adults experienced an increase in loneliness initially, this appeared to level off by late April 2020.[97] Data about the impact of lockdown-related loneliness and isolation on adolescents and young people are perhaps more concerning, with a review of previous research concluding that there may be long-term mental health consequences for these generations.[98] For these groups, although they are generally more comfortable with the kinds of digital technology that allow virtual connections, virtual interactions seem unlikely to adequately replace the important developmental role of face-to-face interactions, and the pandemic coincides with a particularly crucial stage in their life course.[99]

Beyond age groups, the risks of loneliness and social isolation are, yet again, unevenly distributed when looking at demographic and socioeconomic factors. A UK study that compared predictors of loneliness before and during the COVID-19 pandemic found that, although some risk factors for loneliness were the same as before the pandemic (for example, women and people living alone), younger people and people on low incomes experienced an even greater risk of loneliness than usual, while university/college students emerged as a new risk group.[100] A survey in Canada reached similar conclusions, highlighting young women, those on low incomes, and those living alone as experiencing greater loneliness and mental health challenges during the pandemic.[101] When it comes to the role of technology, wealthier groups are almost inevitably better placed, with greater access to hardware, software and spaces from which to have virtual interactions: research identifies this kind of socioeconomic digital divide across multiple contexts, from Nigeria to New York City.[102,103]

Collateral employment, income and wealth impacts

The unequal collateral damage of lockdowns in terms of employment, income and wealth are discussed at length in Chapter Four. These inequalities are crucial to understand because they underpin so much of the other collateral damage discussed in this chapter, shaping access to housing, greenspace, digital technologies and, in many cases, support for health and wellbeing. Rather than preempt the analysis in Chapter Four, which broadly demonstrates that those who were already economically disadvantaged have been further disadvantaged by the pandemic (while a small elite have benefitted), this short section employs two brief vignettes to illustrate the complex ways in which employment, income and wealth interact with the wider collateral damage described in this chapter.

The first vignette comes from the UK and highlights the complex ways in which existing health and socioeconomic conditions can interact with workplace risks and pandemic-related changes to household income, to create a situation in which there are no good options, especially in countries that do not provide a strong social safety net. The vignette emerged from a study of a UK hospital, which found it was cleaners and porters of intensive care areas who were most at risk of catching COVID-19, being even more vulnerable than the medical staff; a lack of personal protective equipment (PPE) meant this group faced double the risk of infection.[104] Many of these workers were also under financial pressure to continue working through the pandemic, even when they were concerned about the risk for themselves and their families. A recent profile of Karen Smith, a cleaner working in Bradford Royal Infirmary, written by her colleague, epidemiologist and clinician Dr John Wright, highlights the impossible situation facing cleaning staff.[105] Karen felt she had to keep working, financially, especially as her partner, Mal, who had been working as a hospital porter, was required to shield due to a chronic health condition. Unfortunately, Karen caught

COVID-19 in April 2020, and the following month her 80-year-old father-in-law, for whom she had been helping to care (as safely as possible), also contracted the virus. While Karen recovered from the immediate health crisis, but continued to experience long-COVID symptoms, her father-in-law did not, leaving Karen experiencing not only long-term personal health problems and grief, but also guilt:

> 'When I start to think about him the tears come and sometimes I'll be crying almost all day – cleaning and crying. If I'm having a bad day, I won't be able to talk ... The guilt is always there, as I'll never know for sure where he picked it up. Mal's dad didn't set foot out of the door, and so in my head I feel such guilt, because we had to go into the house, we didn't have any choice. I go over it all but it's hard to escape from, because I got it, Mal got it and then his Dad got it. Deep down I think that's what's happened, and it will take time to come to terms with.' (Karen, hospital cleaner, UK, 2021)[106]

What this vignette demonstrates is how existing inequalities in health, income, and housing conditions can interact syndemically with pandemic-induced workplace risks and changes in household income, to create a situation in which collateral damage is almost certain to occur. Minimal state support for families like Karen's meant she was faced with the horrendous choice of either putting her family at risk of insufficient income or at risk of COVID-19.

The second vignette, from research in the US focusing on the experiences of women who had previously experienced gender-based violence or abuse, illustrates the difficulties facing women with limited financial resources trying to leave abusive relationships during the pandemic.[107] As discussed earlier in this chapter, there is evidence that gender-based violence increased across the globe during lockdown. Yet, for women trying to escape abusive situations, the unequal economic impacts (see Chapter Four) seem to be making it harder than ever. In the US study, 18% of the women reported having lost a job since the start of the pandemic, and 42% reported that someone else in their household had either lost a job or had their hours reduced.[108] Losing a job impacts women's financial independence, making it harder to leave abusive situations and increasing the stress on the household. Many of those who still had an option to work reported feeling increased pressure to continue with these jobs, even where they worried that it was dangerous for themselves and/or their children (for example, jobs that risked exposing them to COVID-19 or which reduced their ability to support home-schooling or fully protect children from abusive ex-partners).[109] At the same time, several women reported feeling that the levels of resources available for support were substantially reduced, leaving some women homeless and at further risk of both COVID-19 and abuse:

'Access to resources all but disappeared, became homeless and quarantine happened two weeks later. This shelter did not provide access to community resources, I got a list of housing etc. from an advocate at another shelter. Even so, what places were open did not have any availability.' (Female participant, US, 2020)[110]

What this second vignette demonstrates is that the economic impacts of the pandemic described in Chapter Four cause interacting ripples with other facets of inequality that shape people's lives well beyond the immediacy of job and income loss. For women who have experienced abuse, the loss of financial resources, or the pressure to continue to work despite clear risks, may prove fatal.

Conclusion: reducing collateral damage through politics and policy

The impacts of COVID-19 on the outer-layer of Figure 2.2 – the political and environmental contexts that ultimately shape the other social determinants of health and their distribution – are currently least clear and most open to change. Understanding how change might be achieved at this level is crucial, since it is here that there is an opportunity to shape the fundamental causes of health inequalities and the intricately woven collateral damage of the syndemic pandemic that this chapter portrays. As we discuss in Chapter Five, governments can, and do, make very different political and policy choices about how to protect their populations from the kinds of collateral impact this chapter sets out, for example via their social security systems. Although the pandemic circumstances we all find ourselves in are extremely unusual, these experiences vary hugely by political, environmental and economic context; almost all of the collateral damage discussed in this chapter could be reduced and ameliorated by policies that ensure that people have sufficient resources (many of these policies are discussed in Chapter Five). And so it is perhaps no surprise that, as we discuss in Chapter Six, many actors are now calling for change. We can also see growing popular pressure on governments to respond in ways that do not continue to worsen conditions for those already least well off.[111,112] The questions that remain to be answered are, first, what are governments willing (and able) to do in the context of the huge inequalities that COVID-19 is revealing; and second, how will public support and resources shape the substantial collateral damage the pandemic is wreaking? While progressive social movements and researchers (such as ourselves) hope the pandemic will coalesce ideas and action to create a fairer, more equitable world, research suggests these views are competing with reactionary, capitalist and state actors.[113] There is little doubt that, for almost every country, the outer layer of Figure 2.2 will change as a result of the pandemic, but how exactly this layer changes will shape the world that subsequently emerges. We explore this further in Chapters Five and Six.

FOUR

Pandemic precarity: inequalities in the economic crisis

> The strong do what they can and the weak suffer what they must.
>
> Thucydides, 431 BC

Introduction

This chapter examines the COVID-19 economic crisis, an economic shock of rare and extreme impact. COVID-19 has had a devastating impact on the world economy with huge reductions in productivity and national income, and record levels of unemployment (for example and 5.2 million people filed for unemployment benefit in just one week in April 2020 in the US). It is widely feared that the economic impact will be far greater than that of the global financial crisis of 2007/8, and that it is likely to be worse in depth than the Great Depression of the 1930s. Emerging contemporary data and research from previous recessions suggest that the economic fallout from the COVID-19 pandemic will have huge consequences for health and health inequalities. This chapter will provide an overview of the unequal impacts of COVID-19 in terms of the social and spatial distribution of the economic crisis. It will then use evidence from previous recessions (such as the global financial crisis of 2007/8) to explore the likely unequal health impacts and reflect on the role of social safety nets in preventing them.

An unequal crisis

The impact of COVID-19 on health inequalities will not just be in terms of virus-related infection and mortality, but also in terms of the health consequences of the policy responses undertaken in most countries. Traditional public health surveillance measures of contact tracing and individual quarantine were successfully pursued by some countries (most notably by Australia, South Korea and Germany) as a way of tackling the virus in the early stages. However, most other countries failed to employ this approach successfully, so governments worldwide were eventually forced to implement mass quarantine measures in the form of lockdowns and social distancing. These state-imposed restrictions, usually requiring the government to take on emergency powers, have been implemented to varying levels of severity, but all have in common a significant increase in social isolation and confinement within the home and immediate neighbourhood. The aims of these unprecedented measures are to increase social and physical distancing and thereby reduce the effective reproduction number (eR_0) of the virus to below one. For example, in the UK lockdowns of spring and autumn 2020, individuals were only allowed to leave the home for one of four reasons: shopping for basic necessities, one hour of exercise a day, medical needs, travelling for work purposes.[1]

The immediate pathways through which the COVID-19 emergency lockdowns are likely to have unequal health impacts are multiple. They range from unequal experiences of lockdown (for example, due to job and income loss, overcrowding, urbanity, access to greenspace, key worker roles); how the lockdown itself is shaping the social determinants of health (for example, reduced access to healthcare services for non-COVID-19 reasons as the system is overwhelmed by the pandemic); and inequalities in the immediate health impacts of the lockdown (for example, in mental health and gender-based violence). However, arguably, the longer-term and largest consequences of the 'great lockdown' for health inequalities will be through political and economic pathways.[2] The economic shock of COVID-19 can therefore be seen as part of how the pandemic is acting as a syndemic (see Chapter One): COVID-19, as a disease, was exacerbated by existing inequalities (see Chapter Two); and now, via the economic shock, it is in turn creating new inequalities.

The world economy has been severely impacted by COVID-19, with considerable stock market volatility, oil prices crashed, productivity falling (for example, UK gross domestic production [GDP] fell by over 20% in the first six months of 2020), and record levels of unemployment. This was despite the unprecedented interventions undertaken by some governments and central banks, such as the £300 billion injection by the UK government to support workers and businesses in spring 2020 (explored further in Chapter Five). The pandemic has slowed China's economy, with a predicted loss of at least US$65 billion in the first quarter of 2020. Economists fear that the economic impact will be far greater than the global financial crisis of 2007/8, when unemployment in the US, for example, peaked at 10.6%; the deep recession of the early 1980s, when manufacturing employment decreased substantially; and even the Great Depression of the 1930s, when unemployment in the US peaked at 25%. Indeed, it is predicted that it will lead to the largest recession in 300 years – since the Great Frost of 1709.[3] By the end of 2020, UK national wealth (as measured by GDP) fell by 11%, France by over 9%, Germany by around 6%, and almost 5% in the US.[4] In the UK, 750,000 jobs were lost between March and October 2020, unemployment in the US increased by more than 14 million, from 6.2 million in

February to 20.5 million in May 2020, meaning that 13.0% of the workforce were unemployed.[5] Just like the 1918 influenza pandemic (which also had severe impacts on economic performance and increased poverty rates),[6] the COVID-19 crisis will have huge economic, social and, ultimately, health consequences as a result of the ensuing economic recession.

These impacts, though, are unlikely to be experienced equally.[7] Already, there is evidence that the economic shock from COVID-19 has had a disproportionate impact on people with lower educational qualifications, those who already earned less, on younger people, on racial/ethnic minorities, and on women. The US provides a clear example of these economic inequalities.[8] Unemployment rates in May 2020 in the US were significantly lower among workers with higher levels of education: graduate unemployment rates were around 7% compared to over 18% for those with no qualifications. Likewise, the unemployment rate among those aged 16 to 24 in May 2020 was over 25%, more than double that of workers aged 35 and older (which was around 10%). This reflects the concentration of younger and lower-qualified workers in industries, such as retail and hospitality, that were more impacted by social distancing and lockdowns. The US also demonstrates large inequalities in unemployment by race/ethnicity, with the highest unemployment rates in May 2020 found among Hispanic (19.5%) and Black women (17.2%), and Hispanic (15.5%) and Black men (15.8%) (see Table 4.1). Again, this probably reflects that Hispanic and Black Americans are more likely to be employed in those industries most impacted by COVID-19, and in less secure roles. Further, the unemployment rate in the US for all women in May 2020 (14.3%) was higher than the unemployment rate for all men (11.9%). This is potentially because women accounted for the majority of workers in the leisure and hospitality sector and the educational services sector, which were most impacted by the lockdowns and social distancing measures. It might

Table 4.1: Changes in unemployment rates by race/ethnicity and gender in the US (February and May 2020)

Group	Unemployment rate (% of workforce) February 2020	Unemployment rate (% of workforce) May 2020
Black women	5.2	17.2
Hispanic women	5.5	19.5
White women	2.5	11.9
Black men	7.3	15.8
Hispanic men	4.3	15.5
White men	3.5	9.7

Source: Pew Research Center, 2020.

also reflect the fact that women were more likely to take on childcare labour within the home as a result of school closures.

Meanwhile, the wealth of billionaires globally climbed by over a quarter (27.5%), reaching US$10.2 trillion by August 2020, up from US$8.0 trillion at the beginning of April 2020.[9] This was largely a result of these individuals using some of their existing wealth to 'bet' on the recovery of particular firms. This marks a new high for the wealth of billionaires, and signals a further widening of the gap separating those who struggle to cover the basic costs of living and those who have accumulated enough wealth to live the most luxurious lives imaginable multiple times over.

Evidence from England suggests that these COVID-19 increases in unemployment are also unevenly distributed in terms of geography: higher in more deprived towns, cities and regions. For example, analysis by the Northern Health Sciences Alliance found that by April 2020, northern cities in England including Manchester, Liverpool, and Newcastle all experienced above average increases in the rate of people claiming unemployment benefits.[10] Similarly, a report by the Communities in Control association estimated that neighbourhoods with the highest unemployment pre-COVID would suffer the greatest increases in unemployment post-COVID: neighbourhoods where over 15% of the working-age population were already unemployed pre-COVID could see increases of up to 27.5% during 2021.[11] As a result, the Institute for Public Policy Research estimated that by 2021 there will be an additional 300,000 children and 1.7 million adults falling into poverty in England.[12]

Interviews with teachers in England, conducted in April and May 2020 (five to six weeks after most schools closed for the first lockdown) were already picking up on some of these consequences, with some teachers reporting that they had gotten involved in delivering food to the families most in need:

> When you deliver a bag of food to a family who ... literally have nothing ... they have lost their jobs because they were zero hours contract workers; they've got three or four children; and we know on a daily basis when they're in school those children are hungry all the time because we see them ... it ... remind[s] you about society. (Teacher, UK, 2020)[13]

The teachers also noted that the inequalities and poverty they were witnessing were not caused by the pandemic but rather shining a spotlight on, and exacerbating, social inequalities that had already existed. In our words, they were witnessing a syndemic of inequality and COVID-19.[14]

International analysis suggests that the unequal economic impacts evident within the US and UK are not unusual. Moreover, given preexisting differences in government resources, responses to COVID-19, social protection and the economic profile of countries, the economic impacts will vary substantially between countries, as well as within them. Early analysis of data from 32 sub-Saharan African countries, for example, suggests 9.1% of the population immediately fell into extreme poverty as a result of COVID-19 and associated lockdown measures, with the impacts greatest for those already close to the poverty line, single-mother households, and young children.[15] As a result, 31.8 million people, including 3.9 million children under five, became very severely food-deprived,[16] and the UN has warned that several African countries are now facing a hunger pandemic.[17] This was powerfully reflected in the following account of a trader in Benin City, Nigeria (a designated hunger hotspot), who contrasted coronavirus with the 'hunger virus':

'What good is it asking us to stay indoors when we are dying of hunger and no money for us? Does [the] government want us to feed on ourselves? This sickness [COVID-19] is nothing compared to the hunger virus that my children and I face ... I am a widow, I have no support from anyone.' (Benin city trader, 2020)[18]

These unequal increases in unemployment and poverty will have important implications for health inequalities in the medium and longer term; probably more so than the inequalities in COVID-19 itself (see Chapter Two).

Recessions, health and inequality[19]

National economic wealth (that is, GDP) has long been considered the major global determinant of population health, with the vast differences in mortality between high (for example, UK, US, Europe) and low and middle-income countries (for example, India, Ethiopia, Ecuador) accounted for by differences in economic growth.[20] Changes in the economy therefore potentially have important implications for population health and inequalities in health. Recessions are globally defined as two successive quarters of negative growth in GDP.[21] They are characterised by instability (in terms of inflation and interest rates) and sudden reductions in production and consumption, with corresponding increases in business closures and unemployment. For example, the financial crisis of 2007/8 was characterised by peaks in unemployment rates of around 8.5% in the UK and the US, 10% in France and more than 20% in Spain. This economic downturn is popularly referred to as the Global Financial Crisis (GFC) as it was longer, wider and deeper than previous post-war economic downturns, and the worst since the Great Depression of the 1930s. Indeed, high-income economies had not returned to pre-2008 levels of growth before the COVID-19 pandemic hit.

The short-term overall population health effects of recessions are rather mixed, with the majority of international studies concluding that all-cause mortality, deaths from cardiovascular disease and from motor vehicle accidents and hazardous health behaviours *decrease* during economic downturns, while deaths from suicides, rates of mental ill health and chronic illnesses *increase*.[22] Studies suggesting that recessions are 'good for health' have found that mortality rates actually rise during periods of economic growth.[23] For example, a study of mortality trends in the US found that the overall decline in mortality rates in the 20th century actually reversed during periods of recession.[24] One potential explanation of this inverse relationship between mortality rates and recession is that higher unemployment rates lead to a decrease in business activity and therefore a reduction in work-related deaths, combined with a reduction in alcohol and tobacco consumption as incomes decline, resulting in a reduction in mortality risks.[25] Studies have also found that road traffic accidents decrease during periods of recession, as people have less need to drive, and are less able to afford to do so.[26]

In contrast, in terms of mental illness, research suggests that recessions can also be 'bad for health'. For instance, a study found that the mental health of men in England deteriorated over the two years following the GFC recession.[27] Mental health problems such as stress and depression were also found to increase during periods of recession in studies in Spain,[28] Greece[29] and Northern Ireland.[30] There is also evidence of increases in poor mental health and wellbeing after the GFC, including self-harm and psychiatric morbidity.[31,32] In a number of studies this was found to lead to an increase in mortality rates during periods of recession, particularly from suicide.[33] For example, following the 2007/8 crisis, worldwide an excess of 4884 suicides were observed in 2009, and over the next three years (2008 to 2010) an excess of 4750 suicides occurred in the US, 1000 in England, and 680 in Spain.[34] However, it is not just mental health that is negatively affected by recessions, as a number of studies worldwide have found that general health indicators also worsen during times of recession.[35]

One of the main pathways whereby recession affects health is through the adverse impact of unemployment on health. Unemployment is associated with worse mental health, including suicide.[36] It has also been linked to higher rates of all-cause mortality and limiting long-term illnesses,[37] and, in some studies, a higher prevalence of risky health behaviours (particularly among young men), including problematic alcohol use and smoking.[38] Local rates of unemployment are associated with poorer neighbourhood health, and at the country level, increases in the unemployment rate have been associated with increased mortality.[39] Studies from various countries have identified poverty as an important intermediary factor in the relationship between unemployment and health.[40] Indeed, the health gap between employed and unemployed people is lower in countries with more generous benefits for those out of work.[41]

Some studies of previous economic downturns (including those in the 1970s, 1980s and 1990s, as well as the GFC of 2007/8) suggest that the unemployment, and therefore health, effects of economic downturns can be unequally distributed, thereby exacerbating health inequalities.[42] For example, a study in Japan found that economic downturns increased occupational inequalities in general health among men.[43] Further, after the GFC, areas of the UK with higher unemployment rates had greater increases in suicide rates.[44] However, studies have found that recessions do not increase health inequalities in all countries. For example, a Finnish study found that the economic downturn of the 1990s slowed down the trend towards increased socioeconomic inequalities in mortality.[45] Similarly, studies of morbidity conducted in Finland,[46] Norway,[47] Sweden[48] and Denmark[49] found that socioeconomic inequalities in general health remained stable in these countries during the 1980s and 1990s, a period marked by economic volatility and recessions.[50] Similarly, a comparative study of trends in general health from 1991 to 2010 found that there was a more negative impact on the health of those in the lowest educational groups in England, particularly low-educated women, than in Sweden during the recessions of the 1990s and the GFC.[51] These findings are also supported by a study of inequalities in preterm births in the Scandinavian countries, which remained broadly stable from 1981 to 2000 despite periods of economic downturn.[52]

The health inequalities effects of recessions may well, therefore, be experienced quite differently by otherwise similar people and communities, due to national policy variations: more generous welfare systems protect the health of the population and especially the most vulnerable.[53] For example, although early analysis of data in South Africa found that the wages of lower-educated groups have been impacted by COVID-19 more than the wages of higher-educated groups, the financial support provided by the state for poorer households means that the overall impact on household income is actually relatively less for lower-educated households than it is for those with higher levels of education.[54] In sum, intervention by the state is protecting the poorer households, at least to a degree. Analysis of previous economic downturns suggests that the welfare states in social democratic countries (Denmark, Finland, Norway, Sweden) are particularly good at preventing the deterioration of health of the most vulnerable groups during economic downturns.[55] This may be because the comparatively strong social safety nets they provide buffer against the structural pressures towards widening income and health inequalities.[56] The nature of how governments respond, economically and in terms of social and health policy, to the COVID-19 economic crisis is likely to be very important in terms of the effects it has on health inequalities.

This is explored further in the next section, which draws lessons for today from what we know about the health effects of the austerity policies implemented in some parts of Europe after the GFC, and further still in Chapter Five.

Lessons from the global financial crisis: social security nets matter

The welfare state, including the social security system (for example, welfare benefits provided to support people experiencing poverty, unemployment, old age, ill health and so on), housing provision, education and the public healthcare system (for example, the National Health Service), is a key moderator of the social determinants of health.[57] For example, the association between being unemployed and having poorer health is moderated by the level of unemployment benefits that a country pays to their citizens when they experience unemployment.[58] Similarly, there are variations in rates of income received for people out of work due to ill health (sickness/disability benefits), the provision of housing and so forth. Researchers therefore divide welfare systems in high-income countries into different types (discussed further in Chapter Five) on the basis of the generosity of the benefits provided (for example, the value of unemployment benefits compared to average wages); the population covered by the systems (the number of people entitled to receive the benefits); and the rules in place for those when in receipt (for example, sanctions or work requirements).[59]

Studies show that countries with more extensive welfare systems and universal healthcare provision have better health outcomes.[60] For example, they have lower infant mortality rates (IMR), lower overall mortality rates, less mortality at younger ages and, albeit to a lesser extent, increased life expectancy at birth.[61,62,63] Indeed, one study found that the type of welfare state accounted for 20% of the difference in IMR between wealthy countries and 10% of differences in low birth weight babies (LBW).[64] Generous basic state pensions decrease excess mortality in older groups.[65] A comparative analysis found that if the US had the same welfare state generosity as other high-income countries then the average life expectancy in America would be almost four years higher.[66] Currently, however, the US has only a limited social safety net, meaning that state-run and voluntary organisations involved in the provision of food, shelter and basic healthcare have quickly become overwhelmed during the COVID-19 pandemic.[67] A study examining the experiences of those on the frontline of these kinds of basic social services highlights these pressures, with one food bank administrator in Houston, Texas noting that they faced both a greater need for food and a reduced number of volunteers, with dire consequences: 'If you don't have the volunteers to sort and pack the food, the food can't get out the door.'[68]

The importance of social safety nets for health and health inequalities, particularly in times of economic crisis and high unemployment, is exemplified when looking at the impacts of austerity. The GFC of 2007/8 was a result of problems in the US mortgage market, which led to a massive collapse in financial markets across the world. Banks increasingly required state bailouts (for example, in the UK the retail bank Northern Rock was nationalised, while in the US the Lehmann Brothers investment bank filed for bankruptcy and the mortgage companies Freddie Mac and Fannie Mae were given major government bailouts). Stock markets posted massive falls which continued as the effects in the 'real' economy began to be felt, with unemployment rates of over 10% in the US and the eurozone. In 2009, the International Monetary Fund (IMF) announced that the global economy was experiencing its worst period for 60 years.[69] The global economic recession continued throughout 2009 and 2010, and while many wealthy governments injected liquidity into their economies (via so-called quantitative easing), youth unemployment remained high across Europe, particularly in the periphery economies of the eurozone, with rates of over 40% (Greece and Spain) and over 30% (Italy and Portugal). General unemployment levels in Greece amounted to 25% of those aged 16 to 65 in 2015, while poverty rates doubled from rates before the GFC of 2007/8, to 40%. Government debt stood at 177% of GDP in 2015.[70] International creditors pressured the Greek government into substantially reducing public spending in response, requiring a programme of austerity.[71] Hence, alongside the loss of (employment-linked) healthcare facing the millions of Greeks who lost their jobs, public funding for healthcare was simultaneously being reduced, leaving millions without comprehensive health coverage.[72]

Unlike previous recent recessions of the 1980s and 1990s, the GFC was accompanied in many European countries (including the UK, but most notably in Greece and Spain) by escalating public expenditure cuts.[73] Austerity, the practice of reducing budget deficits in economic downturns by decreasing public expenditure and/or increasing taxes, arguably exacerbated the recession in some European countries, most notably in Greece, Spain, Italy and Portugal. The UK, while not as affected as the eurozone by the financial crisis and subsequent recession, still embarked on a programme of austerity. Here, no time was wasted in 'making the most of a crisis', with the 2010–2015 Coalition government (of Conservatives and Liberal Democrats) and then the Conservative government elected in 2015 (and re-elected in 2017 and 2019) enacting large-scale cuts to central and local government budgets, capping NHS budgets, and enacting steep reductions in welfare services and benefits.[74]

It is estimated that the UK welfare reforms undertaken up to 2017 took nearly £19 billion a year out of the economy. This is equivalent to around £470 a year for every adult of working age in the country. However, despite claims at the time by the UK Prime Minister David Cameron that 'we are all in it together', the financial impact of the welfare reforms varied greatly across the country. Professors Tina Beatty and Steven Fothergill of Sheffield Hallam University found that austerity widened the gaps in prosperity between the best and worst local economies across England, increasing the socioeconomic divide between the most and least deprived areas of towns and cities and between richer and poorer parts of the country.[75] Britain's older industrial areas, a number of seaside towns, and some London boroughs, were hit hardest. Much of the south and east of England (outside London) escaped comparatively unscathed. Up to 2015, Blackpool, in the northwest of England, was hit worst of all: an estimated loss of more than £900 a year for every adult of working age in the town. The three regions of northern England lost around £5.2 billion a year in benefit income by 2017. More than two-thirds of the 50 local authority districts worst affected by the reforms were in the northern 'old industrial areas': places like Liverpool, Middlesbrough, Burnley and Sheffield. The higher reliance on benefits and tax credits in northern, post-industrial parts of England meant that austerity had a greater impact here.[76]

Local government spending (excluding police, schools, housing benefit, public health) fell by nearly 30% in real terms between 2008 and 2015 in England. In terms of the geographies of local authority budget cuts, a similar pattern to welfare reform emerges: as a general rule, the more deprived the local authority, the greater the financial hit.[77] At the extremes, the worst-hit local authority areas, mainly located in the north (for example, Middlesbrough), lost around ten times as much, per adult of working age, as the authorities least affected by the cuts, found exclusively in the south and east of England (for example, Hart, Hampshire). Here the cuts amounted to less than £50 per head in this period. In contrast, the loss per working age adult in the worst affected northern districts was £470 a year.

These 'reforms' also disproportionately impacted low-income households of working age and children.[78] In contrast, pensioner households were protected from austerity by, for example, the universal state pension 'triple lock' (a guarantee to increase the state pension every year by the higher of inflation, average earnings, or a minimum of 2.5%), and other universal allowances for the elderly such as the winter fuel allowance.[79] As a result, child poverty rates increased substantially during austerity.[80] Today, child poverty rates in England average 30%; they are highest in the more deprived northern areas with, for example, rates now as high as 41% in Middlesbrough and 39% in Newcastle in the northeast.[81] Indeed, one of the symbols of austerity in Britain was the rise of emergency food banks, largely unknown before 2010 but now with over a million people reliant on them to survive every year. By 2019, prior to the pandemic, the UK had more food banks than McDonalds outlets.[82]

Poverty, and child poverty especially, has huge implications for health and wellbeing. Children born in the most deprived areas of England live, on average, for almost ten years less than their counterparts in the most affluent areas, and spend 20 fewer years in good health (so-called healthy life expectancy).[83] Children living in poverty are also much less likely to do well at school; for example, 69% of children from the most affluent neighbourhoods gain five or more GCSEs compared to only 52% from the most deprived neighbourhoods.[84] The following account of a 15-year-old child, Kwame, living in London, collected as part of an international study of food poverty, provides some visceral insights into how experiences of poverty can impact on children's lives and education:

'I was so hungry and that, so … all of a sudden yeah it was like … it was like … it was like I got hit on my belly … like I got stabbed with a knife'. He contrasts his hunger now with how they ate when he was younger: 'Yeah … we used to like eat. But now … we haven't eaten cos my mum's stopped working, not enough food coming ... we have to like cope with it ... and not spend nothing cos like if you do then we're going to struggle even more'. At school, he reports that his belly is always 'rumbling' and hunger leads to a lack of energy. As a result, he falls asleep on the desk, gets into trouble and is falling behind: '... yeah cos I've done a test and I just feel like I'm not progressing. I even know that I'm not progressing'. He says that he has a 'mood sometimes' when he is hungry and doesn't 'have enough energy to talk'. (Kwame, 15, UK, 2020)[85]

In turn, educational attainment is a strong predictor of future health, employment, income and productivity: only 58% of working age adults with GCSE or lower educational level are employed in the UK, compared to more than 80% of those with university degrees.[86] Child poverty also has long-term impacts on the economy, costing over $1 trillion per year in the US and at least £25 billion a year in the UK.[87,88]

Unsurprisingly, given what we know about the social determinants of health (see Chapters One and Two), studies have found that austerity has led to increases in health inequalities.[89] International analysis found that 'austerity kills': those countries (such as Iceland or the US) that responded to the GFC of 2007/8 with an economic stimulus fared much better, particularly in terms of mental health and suicides, than those countries (for example, Spain, Greece or the UK) that pursued a policy of austerity.[90] Weak social protection systems increased the health and social crisis in Europe;[91] those countries that had higher spending on social welfare considerably reduced their suicide rates during the recession.[92] In the UK, it was estimated that the pressures that austerity placed on key social and healthcare services resulted in up to 10,000 additional deaths in 2018 compared to previous years.[93]

Experiential research reveals the direct consequences of these cuts for both frontline staff and service users. For staff involved in providing access to resources and services, austerity not only reduced options for providing support, even where it was clearly needed,[94] but also created additional pressure to meet targets for reducing the number of people receiving benefits. A recent book by Professor Imogen Tyler recounts one former job centre advisor describing how, overnight, she felt her job changed from one of helping people to one involving 'the persecution of vulnerable people'.[95] Unsurprisingly, greater numbers of people came to experience poverty, often struggling to pay for food, heating and housing, with inevitable consequences for their mental, as well as physical, health:

> There's the stress of always worrying are they going to pay me this week? Am I going to be able to pay my bills? Of course in the meantime your rent goes into arrears, your council tax goes into arrears, it has a chain effect. It's relentless ... you go to bed thinking about it and you wake up thinking about it. (Jimmy, 47, UK, 2018)[96]

Austerity also increased health inequalities. The gap in mental health and wellbeing between deprived and affluent areas increased as people living in more deprived areas bore the brunt of rising rates of mental ill health.[97] Regional inequalities also increased, with, for example, greater rates of increase in suicides in the north than the south of England: by 2012 they were 12.4 per 100,000 in the northwest compared to 8.7 per 100,000 in London. Mortality rates among lower-income women have actually increased in some areas of England.[98] Socioeconomically and spatially concentrated increases in unemployment since 2007/8 also led to an increase in inequalities in both morbidity and mortality.[99] Austerity had a disproportionate impact on the health of vulnerable groups, especially those people and families, including children, on the lowest incomes or in receipt of welfare benefits.[100] An international study found similarly that reductions in public spending adversely affected the mental health of disadvantaged social groups.[101]

This is unsurprising given that an international study exploring people's experiences of poverty found that shame was consistently associated with poverty, across contexts as diverse as Uganda, India, China, Pakistan, South Korea, the UK and Norway.[102] Moreover, in each location, this sense of shame (which, while internally felt, was also externally imposed by others, including those from whom help was being sought) affected people's mental health, resulting in withdrawal, self-loathing, despair, depression and thoughts of suicide.[103] The process by which the sense of feeling externally judged and shamed comes to be internalised is powerfully captured in the opening pages of Professor Tyler's book, *Stigma: The Machinery of Inequality*, in which she describes how the substantial reductions in the UK's safety net implemented during austerity were justified via stigmatising political and media discourses, with visceral consequences for those seeking support, such as her friend, Stephanie:

> Stories about 'benefits cheats' seeped incessantly into Stephanie's world; every time she turned on the radio or television or brushed past a rack of newspapers in a shop, she would come across 'things like these people are stealing your taxes', which left her 'thinking that is me they're talking about'. This 'welfare stigma machine' needled Stephanie from every direction: 'It keeps coming, it's relentless, one constant cycle of judgement, like a knife being stuck repeatedly into you'. This unremitting stigma slowly eroded Stephanie's self-esteem. She began to feel that her daughter would be better off without her. She started to regularly self-harm. She became suicidal: 'I stockpiled tablets waiting for the right moment'.[104]

Research highlighting the effects of austerity on health inequalities is in keeping with previous studies of the effects of public sector and welfare state contractions on increases in health inequalities in the UK, US and New Zealand in the 1980s and 1990s. Such prior research confirms that socially and geographically concentrated cuts to the social safety net increase health inequalities. For example, a US study found that inequalities by income and ethnicity in premature mortality (deaths under age 75) and infant mortality rates (deaths before age one) decreased between 1966 and 1980, and then increased between 1980 and 2002.[105] The reductions in inequalities (1966 to 1980) occurred during a period of welfare state and healthcare coverage expansion in the US (the 'War on Poverty'), and the enactment of civil rights legislation which increased access for African Americans. The increase in health inequalities occurred during the Reagan–Bush period[106] when public welfare services (including healthcare insurance coverage) were cut, funding of social assistance was reduced, the minimum wage was frozen, and the tax base was shifted from the rich to the poor, leading to increased income polarisation.[107]

These findings are mirrored in studies of welfare state reductions in New Zealand which found that socioeconomic inequalities in all-cause mortality increased in the 1980s and the 1990s then stabilised in the early 2000s.[108] Geographical inequalities in health between local areas and regions also increased.[109] The increases in health inequality occurred during a period in which New Zealand underwent major structural reform, including a shift towards a less redistributive tax system; targeted social benefits; privatisation of major utilities and public housing; the introduction of a regressive tax on consumption and user charges for welfare services; and deregulation of the labour market. The stabilisation of inequalities in mortality in the late 1990s and early 2000s occurred during a period in which the economy improved and there were some improvements in services (for example, better access to social housing, more generous social assistance, and a decrease in healthcare costs).

UK research into the health effects of Thatcherism (1979 to 1990) has also concluded that the large-scale dismantling of the UK's social democratic institutions, and the early pursuit of 'austerity-style' policies, increased socioeconomic health inequalities in the 1980s. Thatcherism deregulated the labour and financial markets; privatised utilities and state enterprises; restricted social housing; curtailed trade union rights; marketised the public sector; significantly cut the social wage via welfare state retrenchment; accepted mass unemployment; and implemented large tax cuts for the business sector and the most affluent.[110] In this period, while life expectancy increased and mortality rates decreased for all social groups, the increases were greater and more rapid among the highest social groups so that inequalities increased. Geographical inequalities in health also increased in this period, with the north, parts of Wales and Scotland falling behind the rest of the UK. In these areas, many communities experienced the closure of multiple large employers, and these changes not only threatened people's individual livelihoods and incomes but had multiplicative impacts on whole communities, as the following Welsh valleys resident recounts:

Well the first link to go was the mines. But that was ok after a while, it was devastating for the miners. That was ok really because then some of 'em could get work here. In the steelworks. Some people moved away but a lot of 'em came back as well. A lot of the miners came back and the second chain, the second link in the chain was British Steel. When it was announced it was closing. And to me that was a death knell in the town. And everybody stood still, oh my god. And it was like, if that chain was broken and it was flung away and everybody just, they just didn't know what to do, none of us really. ('Martha', a woman in her 60s, Wales, 2010)[111]

As particular places came to be known as areas of low employment and poverty, stigmatising discourses became associated with those places and residents, in turn, came to feel labelled by the places they lived. Studies exploring people's own accounts of these processes make clear that those who have experienced this know all too well the negative health impacts that can follow,[112] as the following participant in a Scottish study of an area subject to both the 1980s deindustrialisation and the more recent process of austerity reflects:

> I live in Whitecrook and Whitecrook's got a very bad name. It embarrasses my wife tae have tae live there, y'know. She feels embarrassed if she tells people or people have tae come tae the house. It's a shame. It affects her mentally. It affects me tae a slight extent but not as bad, I think the wife's more affected by it. (Owen, photovoice participant Scotland, 2015)[113]

Conclusion

This chapter has examined the syndemic nature of the COVID-19 pandemic by focusing on the inequalities that are emerging from the economic crisis. It has outlined some of the unequal impacts of the economic crisis, including higher unemployment rates in more deprived areas and among the young, women, ethnic minorities and lower-income workers. It has drawn on research into the health effects of previous economic downturns, from the 1980s, 1990s, and the GFC, to outline the likely negative impact on health inequalities. Drawing on research into the effects of the GFC on health inequalities, the chapter has also shown that the unequal health effects are exacerbated by austerity and related cuts to the social safety net. More broadly, the chapter has noted the importance for health inequalities of social security, which protects the health of the most vulnerable parts of society. The COVID-19 pandemic is acting as a syndemic, itself exacerbated by existing inequalities and in turn producing new ones. However, the impact of the economic crisis on health inequalities can be minimised by investments in social safety nets. But the COVID-19 recession does not have to have harmful impacts on health inequalities – our political and policy responses matter for what happens to health inequalities post-COVID-19. This theme is explored further in the next chapter.

FIVE

Pandemic politics: inequality through public policy

Rara avis in terris nigroque simillima cygno.

[A rare bird upon the earth and very much like a black swan.]

Juvenal, AD 100

Syndemic pandemic: black swan, white swan, or grey rhino?

In the second century CE, Roman poet Juvenal likened finding the perfect woman to seeing a black swan in the wild: both were considered so unlikely as to be impossible. But after Dutch navigator Willem de Vlamingh encountered a swan with all black feathers while exploring southwestern Australia in 1697, the black swan instead became a metaphor for erroneously assuming that something is impossible based on the limited facts at one's disposal – in this case, the observation that in Europe, all swans were white. By 2020, 'black swan' had come to symbolise for market investors an event with serious effects that is nevertheless so rare as to be unpredictable, based on the current state of knowledge.[1] So when the Silicon Valley venture capital firm Sequoia Capital referred to the COVID-19 pandemic as a 'black swan' in a memo issued on 5 March 2020,[2] everyone knew what they meant: something terrible and unpredictable had happened, and all we could do now was figure out how to deal with the consequences.

But, much like the actual black swan 'discovered' by Willem de Vlamingh, COVID-19 was quite predictable to those who were paying attention to all of the available facts. Scientists had been warning for decades that the combination of climate change and human encroachment on natural habitat made it not only possible but likely that a pandemic disease would cross over from an animal population to humans.[3,4,5] The spread of SARS, MERS, Ebola, swine flu, avian flu and Zika should all have prepared us for this possibility. If anything, the COVID-19 pandemic was a white swan, not a black one.

The threat of growing inequities resulting from COVID-19, on the other hand, was more like a 'gray rhino', a metaphor coined by strategist Michele Wucker: that is, a threat that is predictable – not to say obvious – in light of existing warnings and visible evidence; is quite dangerous; and is also avoidable.[6] When a two-ton animal is stomping its feet and threatening to charge, there is still time to get out of the way, even if the moment for preventing its anger has already passed. And this is the situation that confronted governments when the COVID-19 pandemic hit. There was nothing they could do at that point to prevent the emergence of a novel coronavirus with pandemic potential, and it was too late to do anything substantial to abate the impact of preexisting social inequalities on people's health as the disease struck. These preexisting inequalities were the product of earlier political choices about the acceptable level of inequality in society. However, governments *could* act to prevent even greater inequalities from arising out of the pandemic.

Some governments did a great deal to try to reduce the unequal impacts of COVID-19 on their populations, while others did far less. And it turned out that in places where there were already higher levels of social protection and less inequality prior to the pandemic, governments also acted most forcefully to prevent new inequalities arising.

This tells us that the syndemic nature of the pandemic is not a fact of nature, but of politics: the syndemic of inequality and COVID-19 was less intense where governments had already decided to act to reduce inequality before the pandemic; and where they decided to do more to reduce social inequalities during the pandemic.

In this chapter, we consider the politics behind the current syndemic that the previous chapters have outlined. We focus on high-income, democratic countries in North America, Australasia and Europe, all of which have state-funded systems of welfare or social security intended to ensure citizens' basic needs are provided for. For a global pandemic, this represents a relatively narrow focus but, by honing in on these relatively comparable contexts, we gain a much clearer view about the role that political choices play.

Three worlds of inequality

We have already seen in Chapter One that inequalities in health are related to inequalities in income and social conditions. But where do these latter inequalities come from? The world before the pandemic was not an equal one: even in the rich, industrialised democracies, many people lacked access to the financial and social resources they needed to live healthy lives. But the extent of inequality of circumstances and of health differed between even the quite similar countries of Europe and North America, in ways that would affect how the pandemic played out and the kinds of new inequalities that it created. This section of the chapter discusses the political choices and the public policies that produced these pre-pandemic inequalities.

Most of us know that some countries are more equal than others. Many people also have a perception that the Nordic countries are the most equal, and the English-speaking countries the least equal, of the world's rich democracies. This perception is by and large correct, although with some caveats. If we look across the scope of the late 20th century and into the early 21st, the countries with the smallest inequalities in income among their citizens are those found in the northwest of Europe (including the Nordic countries and the Netherlands), while the UK, the US, Ireland, and Australia have the largest socioeconomic inequalities. Most of the countries of continental western Europe have occupied a middle zone, with somewhat higher inequality in income and social conditions in southern Europe than in the north of the continent. Inequality has been increasing very rapidly in most of the Nordic countries since the 1990s, albeit from a low baseline, and has spiked in both southern Europe and the UK since the GFC of 2008 to 2010. However, the rest of the continent has experienced more moderate growth in inequality, leading to something of a convergence among countries in recent years around a higher overall level of inequality.[7]

Even so, there remain significant enough differences among countries in their general level of economic inequality that it is possible to speak of three types of countries that, because of similarities in their political systems and policy choices, have similar levels of social and labour market protection for their residents. As a result, the countries within each of these three groups also experience similar levels of social inequality, and ultimately similar levels of health inequality.[8]

In 1990, the Danish sociologist Gøsta Esping-Andersen described three 'worlds' of welfare capitalism, based on patterns of politics and policy that are still visible to this day.[9] In the *social-democratic* world, comprising the Nordic countries and the Netherlands, working- and middle-class voters united behind large ruling social-democratic parties that worked to provide generous social policies available to all, labour market policies focused on full employment and high worker productivity, and to prioritise relatively low levels of income inequality. A second, *corporatist* world of welfare, exemplified by most of the countries of continental western Europe and built up after World War Two by a combination of center-right and center-left governments, provided generous social benefits for the core (generally male) workforce, but at the cost of higher unemployment and greater earnings inequality. In the third, *liberal*, mainly English-speaking world, political parties inspired in part by free-market ideologies oversaw much of the construction of the welfare state, resulting in policies that did less to reduce income inequality.

These three different approaches to welfare and inequality resulted in differences in health inequalities before the pandemic, for the reasons laid out in Chapter One. Social-democratic welfare states, which had the lowest overall levels of social inequality, also tended to have better health outcomes for those at the top and those at the bottom of the socioeconomic ladder: more equal countries almost always do better in social and health outcomes.[10] Health inequalities were somewhat larger on average in the corporatist welfare world, corresponding to larger socioeconomic inequalities. And despite the fact that some of the liberal welfare states, like the UK and Canada, had robust, well-funded universal healthcare systems, these countries joined the other members of the liberal world in having especially large and intractable health inequalities, resulting from large and intractable socioeconomic inequalities.

How political policy choices affected pandemic inequalities

As we saw in Chapters Two, Three and Four, COVID-19 has hit unequally everywhere, because of the syndemic link with social inequality, which exists everywhere albeit to different extents. We don't yet know precisely what the size and shape of inequalities in COVID-19 will be in different countries, but we can begin to make some educated guesses. Some of the policies that were characteristic of different welfare worlds *before* the pandemic also likely played an important role in shaping the health inequalities that emerged *during* the pandemic, protecting groups that were at high risk from even greater harm.

For example, the social-democratic and corporatist welfare worlds both tend to have generous paid sick leave for employees. In the liberal world, however, weaker sickness protections for (especially lower-paid, lower-status) workers have long meant that those who fall ill must choose between endangering themselves and others by going to work, or losing their jobs and their income.[11]

Research on young adults living in some of England's poorest northern areas highlights precisely this tension for citizens of liberal welfare worlds. Reflecting on the type of work the young people they interviewed described, Professors Robert MacDonald and Tracy Shildrick write: 'This was not employment that was based on terms and conditions, formal or informal, or which was notable for the fair or compassionate treatment of workers (for example, paid sick leave was rarely available). They worked for employers who were as quick to fire as they were to hire.'[12] A recent book exploring workplace presenteeism notes that, in the US, the situation is even worse: prior to the pandemic, one in five jobs in the US were held by worker contract, meaning there was no sick pay for those who were too ill to work, with the unsurprising result that many continued to show up to work despite being ill.[13] In normal times, this is a matter of concern for those affected; in a global pandemic of a highly transmissible virus, this quickly becomes a concern for everyone.

While most governments eventually put into place emergency measures that protected the livelihoods of workers who stayed home due to infection with SARS-Cov-2, liberal states (most notably the US) that did not already have such protections were less prepared to do so and failed to contain the growth of the pandemic in the early days and weeks.

In countries where strict lockdowns eventually occurred (including most of the corporatist welfare states), all except essential workers were forced to stay home. But where lockdowns did not occur, and avoiding workplaces and transit was made theoretically optional, stronger pre-pandemic protections for workers and citizens were what made it possible for people, especially those with lower incomes and less prestigious jobs, to exercise the option to avoid exposure and potential infection by staying home. This is likely one reason why infection rates were consistently much higher in the liberal UK and US than in social-democratic Denmark or Norway, despite the fact that none of those countries imposed strict lockdowns. In addition to paid sick leave, policies common in the social-democratic welfare world – generous income replacement for those unable to work and guarantees that housing, healthcare, and childcare will be affordable even to those on reduced incomes – made it possible for more people to stay home, self-isolate and stay well. Meanwhile, robust occupational safety measures and strong protections against unfair dismissal meant that fewer essential workers were avoidably put in harm's way.

This difference is clearly evident if we look at the positive accounts of researchers who examined the experiences of nursing home staff in Norway and primary healthcare in Iceland, where changes made in response to COVID-19 were rapid and provided relatively good protection for staff.[14,15] In contrast, accounts detail the concerns of healthcare workers in the UK, where PPE was in short supply during spring 2020:

> I always felt depressed throughout the day as I was fearing to be infected by COVID-19 and in turn take it home to my child who has asthma. (Female mental health nurse, UK, 2020)[16]

> When you walk into work … you don't know what you will find … PPE was running out quickly and you are caught up in between your duty of care and your family safety. (Male healthcare assistant, UK, 2020)[17]

In the corporatist and some of the social-democratic world, many countries experienced strict lockdowns early in the pandemic. However, livelihoods were still put at risk by the sharp economic crisis that the pandemic provoked (see Chapter Four). Many of these countries had preexisting policies that subsidised firms in return for maintaining employment during the period of business contraction: so-called 'short-work' arrangements. Such policies were deployed quickly in Germany and Denmark, for example, blunting some of the immediate impact of the pandemic and protecting incomes. Given the strong, positive relationship between employment, earnings, and health, these policies also likely had the effect of protecting health.

The pre-pandemic configuration of healthcare systems, too, likely made a difference for health outcomes during the pandemic. Most healthcare systems have been subject to intense cost-containment measures since the late 1990s, but in places where health budgets allowed for more intensive care hospital beds and more medical staff per capita, hospitals were better able to accommodate people who needed acute care due to COVID-19 or other conditions.[18,19] Germany, for example, had an average of 29 intensive care unit beds per 100,000 inhabitants, compared to only 10 per 100,000 inhabitants in Spain and 7 in the UK.[20] Similarly, while Germany went into the pandemic with an average of 30 ventilators per 100,000 inhabitants, the UK had only 12 per 100,000 and Spain just 5.[21] While more hospital capacity could be built or nationalised once the pandemic hit, as occurred in the UK and Spain, those countries that already had what in normal times would be 'excess' health system capacity were better able to care for the ill. Hence, as healthcare systems in Italy, Spain, the UK and the US all struggled, with regular reports of hospitals having to stop all non-urgent healthcare work and even turn patients away,[22,23,24] major hospitals in Germany reported being able to continue functioning at full capacity while simultaneously dealing with COVID-19 outbreaks.[25]

Who has access to affordable healthcare provided by welfare states also obviously affected the impact of the pandemic. For example, millions of Americans lack health insurance, or are under-insured, and were thus unable before the pandemic to receive adequate treatment for conditions like diabetes, asthma and cardiovascular disease.[26] These conditions make people who are infected with SARS-Cov-2 more likely to have severe symptoms or die (see Chapter Two). Lack of access to a regular source of healthcare has also made it difficult for uninsured people to get access to COVID-19 tests, resulting in unnecessary spread of the infection. However, it is worth noting that healthcare is one area of social policy that varies in unexpected ways across the three worlds of welfare.[27] For example, the UK's National Health Service, which provides medical care free at the point of service as a right of citizenship, is an unexpected entitlement in a welfare state that is otherwise tolerant of high levels of inequality and less enthusiastic about broad, generous, public welfare programmes. Southern European countries, which in most respects resemble the corporatist welfare states of the northern continent, also have (unexpectedly) chosen to provide access to publicly-provided healthcare as a right of citizenship. Meanwhile, elements of employment-based health insurance make social-democratic Finland, which has the lowest level of income inequality in the world, less equalising in the realm of access to healthcare. However, access to healthcare plays a relatively small role in generating health inequalities compared to the impact of deprivation and the other social determinants of health (see Chapter One).[28] That means that, except in cases like the US, where large numbers of people entirely lack access to affordable healthcare, pre-pandemic health policies are less relevant to the production of health inequalities during the pandemic than are other social policies related to income, employment, housing and the like.

The three distinctive worlds of welfare and inequality grew up because in these groups of countries, different ideas about the appropriate way to manage the economy dominated; the relative power and interests of workers, employers, and the self-employed differed; and national institutions (for example differing types of tax and electoral systems) made certain kinds of policies more or less possible.[29,30] But differences in the level of social inequality that occurred in these different worlds of welfare existed, above all, because of *political choices* about how much inequality to allow. Overall, there has been a trend toward increasing inequality among almost all of these countries since the 1980s, and this too has been a political choice.[31,32] Nevertheless, there are still distinctive differences across countries in the degree to which the most radical neoliberal policy prescriptions have been adopted since the 1980s, resulting in differing levels of social inequality. So if there is one thing to take away from the syndemic inequalities that emerged in the early stages of the pandemic, it is that they were avoidable: previous social policy choices shaped the pandemic by shaping social inequality. And as we shall see, the policies that governments have pursued in the midst of the pandemic are *also* the result of choices: choices about how much inequality we will permit going forward.

Inequalities under lockdown

When the pandemic hit, politicians had a series of choices to make about how to manage the spread of disease. In the early phases of the pandemic, inequality was not on the minds of most policy makers. The most immediate task was simply to make sure that as few people as possible became infected, to flatten the curve of the epidemic so as to avoid overwhelming healthcare services. For example, Italy, the first country outside of China to have a large number of COVID-19 cases, enacted relatively indiscriminate lockdowns in the most heavily affected northern regions, restricting all travel and gatherings, closing businesses, schools, and government offices, and prohibiting most people from leaving their homes. In other countries that had more time to prepare, however, measures undertaken to halt the spread of COVID-19 were often hesitant, partial or delayed, potentially exacerbating the already differential impact on different groups in society. How did this variation in the experience of lockdown affect inequalities? And why did different countries make different choices in response to the initial threat?

It is too early to know definitively how variation in lockdown policies affected inequalities. But there are a few things that we know for sure. First, the way that school and childcare closures were handled was a major source of new inequalities. Most countries did close schools for some amount of time, which of course meant that parents, particularly mothers, of young children also had to cease work or else find alternate childcare arrangements. Where schools and businesses closed and reopened in tandem, there was less additional stress on parents with low incomes. However, in those countries that closed schools while businesses remained open, such as the US, failure to provide parents with time off from work and money to make up for their lost income generated a host of new inequalities. Low-income single-parent families faced impossible choices: should the parent go to work, leaving the child alone and potentially bringing illness back into the home? Or should they quit work, risking hunger and homelessness?

Even activities that were still allowed, such as shopping in grocery stores and pharmacies, became problematic. The following account was shared by a single mother in Canada via an online post on 2 April 2020, and reprinted in an academic essay, written by another single parent, which reflects on precisely these challenges:[33]

If anybody has ever wondered what defeat looks like, here it is folks. This is the look of a single mom during a pandemic. The look of a single mom who hasn't left the house except for a grocery order pickup since they called the State of Emergency … The look of a single mom who decided to pack up the children to go to Costco to pick up a prescription and to hopefully get the rest of the things I needed to be able to stay home for a few weeks at least. Because my options are a) get a babysitter which I'm not allowed to do b), leave the kids home alone which I'm not allowed to do, or c) get someone to pick up my stuff which by the way equaled 300$. So this is the look of a single mom who was rudely told by not one, not two, but three Costco employees that it is the last time I will be able to bring in my children, and overheard two employees rudely point at me and say 'yeah are we putting up signs about children because clearly they're not gonna listen until we do'. Most employees were amazing, smiling, and friendly, but I'm guessing a few stressed ones took it out on me. You're looking at the face of a single mom … who's been trying to follow the rules, who has been trying my best at working from home with an eight-year-old and a four-year old who fight and scream and need to eat and are bored just like every other kid. And the look of a single mom who came out of Costco with tears streaming down her face to hear that I will now have to add homeschooling to the mix. (Single mother, Canada, 2020)[34]

In two-earner families, new gender inequalities emerged, as women were overwhelmingly the ones to leave their jobs in order to care for children and supervise remote schooling. An unprecedented number of women in the US, for example, have left the labour market (that is, they are not seeking employment after having been laid off or quitting their jobs, often due to lack of childcare).[35] There is little reason to believe that women are faring better in societies where schools and childcare centres have similarly been closed while large numbers of workers are still expected to show up for their jobs; but governments that prioritised keeping schools open over reopening bars and restaurants, and that made sure childcare was available for essential workers, are less likely to exacerbate the gender and ethnic inequalities that are associated with labour market status.

A second source of inequality in the impact of COVID-19 was the definition and treatment of essential workers during periods of lockdown, both of which varied widely across countries. The segregation of labour markets by gender, race and ethnicity means that in all countries, many of the workers who were labelled 'essential' (nurses and nursing home aides, grocery store clerks, meat packers and farm workers, delivery drivers, transit and sanitation workers) are disproportionately members of racial and ethnic minority groups, often immigrants; and especially in the case of nursing and service-sector workers, also very often women.[36] This is one reason for the striking difference in death rates across racial and ethnic groups early in the pandemic. When the pandemic hit, governments had little choice about the demographic makeup of different segments of the workforce (although prior policies did influence it). But they could control how they defined and treated essential workers, and the extent to which they were exposed to illness and potential death as a result of their status as essential workers. Where the definition of 'essential' was stringent, fewer workers were exposed to the risk of infection in their workplaces and on their commutes; and where protections for essential workers were robust, they were less likely to become ill and better cared for if they did.

Government decisions about whom to declare as essential workers, who could be compelled to work during lockdown periods, clearly had important consequences for inequality. Where businesses were defined as essential merely to ensure continued profitability for their owners, workers suffered unnecessarily. For example, in April 2020 President Trump declared meatpacking plants 'critical infrastructure' and mandated that they remain open to ensure the continuity in the US meat supply – but did not halt exports of pork and chicken to China, despite mounting evidence that meatpacking plants were COVID-19 hotspots. As of October of 2020, more than 44,000 US meatpacking workers had tested positive for COVID-19.[37] Governments made other choices, too: where money for hiring extra workers to fill in for people who fell ill was made available, essential workers could avoid working double and triple shifts that exposed them to the virus for longer periods of time each day. Where governments secured adequate production of PPE, such as masks and gloves, and mandated that employers of essential workers provide it at no cost, these workers were better protected. All of these choices likely led to differences in the number of COVID-19 cases and death among essential workers, which also contributed to gender and racial/ethnic inequalities in the effects of the pandemic.

As for why these policies varied, in some cases the response was likely idiosyncratic and ideological; that is, rather than reflecting longstanding patterns of public policy, government policy was up to how individual leaders decided, in a moment of extreme crisis, to handle the COVID-19 outbreaks that they saw appearing in their own countries. But the patterning of policy responses across countries suggests that there was more to these choices than essentially random decisions by individual leaders. During periods of lockdown, essential workers in the social-democratic welfare world tended to be narrowly defined; to benefit from strict regulation of working conditions and ample provision of PPE to protect them from the virus; to receive generous protection from income loss if they did contract COVID-19; and to be eligible for enhanced childcare and mental health services to ease the burden on their families. In the corporatist welfare states, protection for essential workers was more variable: stronger in some countries (for example, Germany) than in others (for example, France); and stronger for some sectors (for example, public services) than others (for example, food production). In the liberal welfare world, more people tended to fall into the categories deemed essential, and protections for these workers were weaker. These differences in policies are so stark that even at this early date, it seems clear that political choices during the pandemic about when and how to lock down economies, and what social supports would be available, are likely to affect the magnitude of COVID-19 inequalities across different countries and worlds of welfare.

Variation in political and policy responses to the pandemic

Because social policies in a variety of sectors (including but not limited to healthcare) play such an important role in structuring health inequalities (Chapters One to Four), there is every reason to expect that what governments chose to do (or not do) in these areas during the pandemic will have an important impact on the health inequalities that emerge during and after the pandemic. This section describes the very different social policy responses to the health, social, and economic challenges of the pandemic across countries. From labour market policy to childcare to the hospital sector, how governments chose to respond to the crisis has a direct bearing on how unequal the pandemic will be.

Just as countries varied in their immediate response to the emerging pandemic (for example, in the timing and stringency of travel bans and lockdowns, in the scale of testing and contact tracing, and in the decisions about school and business closures), so too did their social policy responses once it became clear that the pandemic would be with us for some time. However, just as government leaders chose from a similar toolkit of emergency response measures, so too did they rely on a similar menu of social policy responses. What varies, then, is not so much the types of things that governments did to help their citizens and their economies through the pandemic; but the scale and scope of these interventions. In other words, the difference is not what's on the menu, but how big the portions are, and who gets to eat at the restaurant! These often reflected preexisting political and policy trajectories. Nearly all governments in the rich, industrialised democracies employed some combination of:

- *direct assistance to citizens to aid with their living costs*, for example, expanded access to cash assistance or tax credits; income replacement during sickness and unemployment; rent assistance; eviction moratoria;
- *supports for private-sector firms*, for example, short-work, shared-work, and subsidised furlough arrangements; subsidies for key business inputs like labour, commercial rents, electricity, and credit; easing regulations such as weekly working time limits and allowing free movement of essential workers; and tax holidays;
- *supports for essential workers*, such as priority access to testing and treatment for COVID-19; workplace safety regulations and PPE to reduce the likelihood of infection; enhanced eligibility for sickness pay; bonuses for hazardous work; and access to childcare and mental healthcare services; and
- *interventions in the healthcare sector*, for example, expanded access to low- or no-cost health services, including universal testing, treatment, and vaccination for COVID-19; measures to secure the supply chain for medical equipment and supplies, including joint purchasing arrangements, centralised inventory management and distribution, and reduced import tariffs on essential medical goods; and efforts to increase health system capacity such as increased funding to local and state health authorities, temporary changes to medical licensure regulations, mobilising the armed forces to assist with logistics, or commandeering private hospital beds for publicly insured COVID-19 patients.

Across the three worlds of welfare, most governments selected some or all of the interventions listed, leading to what at first glance seems to be a similar policy response across countries. However, a closer look reveals important differences and patterns that should by now be familiar to us: The social-democratic world implemented the most generous measures designed to secure universal access to health services, to protect essential workers, and to buoy both household finances and the national economy by activating extensive supports for firms and workers hit by the pandemic-associated economic slowdown. Corporatist welfare states tended to be a bit less universally generous than in the social-democratic world, and interventions in the health sector tended to take a lighter touch. But governments still could and did act as needed, making efforts to ensure that residents had access to healthcare and that most essential workers were supported. Income maintenance programmes were expanded to cover more citizens, and firms were supported through hard economic times using a variety of preexisting policy tools such as short-work arrangements. In the liberal world, meanwhile, social programmes and supports for business and the healthcare sector were also expanded, but from a much lower baseline, in a more patchwork fashion, and in ways that relied more on market mechanisms and personal discretion than on direct government provision or regulation.

Of course, there was also some variation within worlds in the social policy response to the pandemic. For example, French policies were less robust than Germany's, Denmark's response was more inclusive than Sweden's, and even within the UK, Scottish policymakers offered a broader array of supports than that enacted by Westminster. Moreover, the federal political systems in all three of the welfare worlds (for example, Germany, Spain, Canada, and the US) faced unique challenges when confronted with the need for national-level coordination of services such as health and education, which would ordinarily rest mainly in the hands of subnational units. As a result, their responses tended to be different from those in unitary states. Even so, distinctive policy patterns can still be observed in the three worlds of welfare as they responded to the COVID-19 crisis.

How can we explain the persistence of these different basic approaches to social protection across the three worlds of welfare, even when they are confronted with a fundamentally new and global threat? One possible explanation is culture: that is, policymakers and members of the public in the different welfare worlds want their governments to respond in different ways. In this view, the main reason for the lack of generosity or coordination of response in a country such as the US or the UK would be that people just don't want, or expect, their national governments to provide the same level of protection from a threat like COVID-19 as, say, Danish or German people do. There may be an element of truth to the idea that there are national cultures of social protection that tend to prevail even in a crisis, and longstanding political divisions can overlap with social divisions in ways that make it harder to protect certain groups (for example, racial minorities or immigrants). Reinforcing this, as noted in Chapter Four, policy and media sources can construct and promote discourses that frame those in need as undeserving.[38] Nonetheless, it seems far-fetched to believe that democratic majorities anywhere would have supported a limited, ineffective response to the pandemic in favour of a more robust one if they had had the option.

Two other factors likely have more to do with the similarities within worlds of welfare, and differences across them, in their approaches to social policy during the pandemic. First, it is much easier to expand or amend an existing social programme than it is to create a new programme from whole cloth, especially during a period of crisis when administrative resources are stretched thin. This means that countries that already had generous social provisions before the pandemic hit, that is, the social-democratic and corporatist welfare states, were able to respond most rapidly by building on existing programmes; and this is exactly what they did. From social assistance to healthcare to labour markets, governments that already had a high capacity to act to ensure social and economic welfare in most cases used the tools that they had at their disposal, ensuring a relatively timely and robust response that prevented the emergence of new inequalities. For example, it took very little administrative effort for Denmark or Germany to activate and extend their existing short-work programmes, sickness benefits and the like, to prevent the pandemic from worsening existing inequalities. Meanwhile, in countries that had more limited social protection infrastructure in pre-pandemic times, typically in the liberal world, the response to the pandemic was generally weaker, because there was less to build upon and more needed to be created from scratch.

A second, related factor is that governments in the different welfare worlds have tended to rely on different ways of intervening even when they hope to achieve the same goals. For example, while corporatist welfare states would be inclined to act to make sure a low-income family could make ends meet by providing cash assistance, a liberal government would be more likely to offer a tax credit or housing voucher, while a social-democratic welfare state would likely provide low-cost childcare and a place in public housing. When a government is accustomed to using a particular set of policy tools to solve problems – be it direct provision of goods and services, regulation of markets, incentivising behaviours through tax and subsidy regimes, or providing cash benefits – those are the tools they are most likely to reach for in a crisis. This likely explains the disastrous decision of the UK government to circumvent their own public health authorities and contract out testing and contact tracing operations to private actors; as well as more felicitous choices such as the Swedish government's supporting essential workers by expanding publicly provided childcare, or even the European Union's decision to promote extension of unemployment benefits in member states by exempting these payments from the calculation of fiscal shortfalls. Governments responded to the crisis using the tools that were familiar and available, leading to an increase in inequalities in some cases, and in others, to their mitigation.

Given all that is known about the influence of social policies on the social determinants of health (see Chapter One), and on inequality more broadly (see Chapter Four), we can be sure that how governments chose to respond to the pandemic by way of social policy is important for the inequality-COVID-19 syndemic. It's too early to say which interventions in particular might have helped to shape the precise health outcomes of the pandemic in different countries, but we already know a great deal about how social policies are likely to have affected people's ability to cope. The more encompassing and supportive the social policy response was, the more people will have been protected from having to go to work in unsafe conditions, and the fewer will have had to choose between being exposed to illness and feeding, housing and caring for their children. While marginalised groups across societies have suffered the brunt of the health effects of the pandemic (see Chapter Two), universal social policies that protect all inhabitants will have at least given a fighting chance to precarious workers, undocumented migrants, and racial/ethnic minorities. And robust efforts to protect families and firms from economic distress will have buffered the impact of the pandemic on the syndemic inequalities that increase ill health.

Conclusion: pandemic politics

When the COVID-19 pandemic hit, the result was a syndemic of inequality and illness, generated both by pre-pandemic political choices and by policies adopted in the teeth of COVID-19. Politically-created inequalities in society before the pandemic shaped the vulnerability of individuals to the disease; and governments' decisions about what to do during the pandemic shaped the inequalities that would emerge from the pandemic.

Most often, governments acted during the pandemic in ways that reinforced existing patterns of policy and inequality. This is no surprise: politics and policy are very often 'path dependent', meaning that decisions made in the past set the terms of debate for and often constrain the next round of decision making.[39] And this path dependence helps explain why the categorisation of rich democracies into 'three worlds' of welfare by Esping-Andersen in 1990 still does such a good job, 30 years later, of predicting how governments would respond to COVID-19.[40,41]

Even so, some governments have strayed from the paths indicated by their basic welfare institutions, and made choices that resulted in experiencing the pandemic in a way that was atypical for their welfare 'world'. Swedish lawmakers, for example, behaved quite differently from their counterparts in neighbouring social-democratic welfare states. While Denmark and Norway acted early to contain the spread of the virus and to ensure the safety of essential workers and their families, the Swedish national government declined to mandate travel bans, lockdowns or curfews, allowed schools and many businesses to remain open, left it up to individuals to adopt social distancing measures, and failed to ensure adequate access to testing and PPE. Some of these decisions, such as the decision not to ban travel across national borders, were based on available evidence about the (in)efficacy of certain interventions in preventing the spread of the disease.[42,43] It is still not fully clear which of these policy decisions, if any, are causally related to the greater difficulty in controlling the spread of COVID-19 and the higher rates of excess mortality experienced in Sweden as compared to neighbouring countries;[44] but the difference in both policies and the impact of COVID-19 is striking and unexpected. Political choices led to policies and, there is reason to think, outcomes that have exacerbated existing health inequalities in Sweden, particularly the excess burden of disease and death among ethnic minorities and elderly people living in group settings.[45]

Variation in the political choices of governments within the liberal world of welfare is even more striking, if less surprising (the UK and, to an even greater extent, the US have long been recognised as outliers even in the liberal welfare world, mainly for their unusually permissive attitude toward inequality).[46,47] US and UK governments led by parties of the political right have consistently failed to adopt policies that could have mitigated the effects of COVID-19 on vulnerable groups and interrupted the self-reinforcing nature of the inequality-pandemic syndemic. Meanwhile, the leaders of more progressive government coalitions from New Zealand to Ireland to Canada have made very different choices in the face of the pandemic. Their decisions – to offer policy support to essential workers; to entrust well-funded public health agencies with robust testing and contact tracing operations; to provide financial assistance to workers at risk of income loss due to stringent lockdowns – have helped not only to control the spread of the disease, but also to lessen its unequal impacts.[48,49,50]

In other words, some governments in the liberal world of welfare were able to do a great deal to reduce the unequal impact of COVID-19 on their populations despite preexisting patterns of policy that were less egalitarian than in other welfare state types. This should serve as a strong reminder that the inequality-COVID-19 syndemic is a chosen destination, not a preordained destiny.

To help us find our way to a more equal future, despite the pandemic, we will need to change not only our policies, but also our politics. Chapter Six summarises many of the policy choices discussed earlier in this book that we have seen can reduce the self-reinforcing downward spiral of inequality and COVID-19. In this final chapter we pay particular attention to policies that can help reinforce more equal outcomes as we emerge from the pandemic. It also invites us to consider changes to our political institutions that could make these policies more likely, by increasing the voice of ordinary people in the policymaking process.

SIX

Conclusion: health and inequality beyond COVID-19

'Hope' is the thing with feathers –
That perches in the soul –
And sings the tune without the words –
And never stops - at all -

Emily Dickinson, 1891

Introduction

This book has documented the unequal impact of the COVID-19 pandemic. It has sought out the causes of the health inequalities that emerged from the pandemic, and located them in the syndemic of social inequality and the novel coronavirus. We have argued that the COVID-19 pandemic is unequal in four ways:

First, *the pandemic is killing unequally* (Chapter Two). In every country that has been affected by the pandemic, more people are ill, and there are more deaths from the disease, in the places where the most deprived people live. There are also significant inequalities across racial and ethnic groups. This is because of the interaction of the pandemic with existing social, economic and health inequalities.

Second, *the pandemic is being experienced unequally* (Chapter Three). Successive lockdowns designed to quickly halt the spread of COVID-19 when case numbers are rising rapidly have resulted in a significant increase in social isolation for nearly everyone; but the social and economic experiences of lockdowns have been unequal. Lower-income workers are more likely to experience job and income loss, live in higher-risk urban and overcrowded environments, and have higher exposure to the virus by occupying key worker roles.

Third, *the pandemic is impoverishing unequally* (Chapter Four). The pandemic has resulted in an unprecedented shock to the economy from which we have yet to emerge. Job losses, wage reductions, higher debt, and more poverty, as well as increases in the 'deaths of despair', are likely to follow, if previous economic downturns are any guide. However, the social and geographical distribution of these economic impacts will be unequal, with low-income workers, women and ethnic minorities once again bearing the brunt.

Fourth, *the pandemic's inequalities are political* (Chapter Five). The unequal impacts of COVID-19 were not inevitable: the pandemic was a predictable event, and the unequal effects could have been, and indeed in some countries were, mitigated or avoided through better preparation. Policymakers in the past made decisions that led to many of the pandemic's unequal impacts in the present, and once the pandemic began made further choices about how to address emerging inequalities. Governments responded differently, and those with higher rates of social inequality and less generous social security systems experienced a more unequal pandemic.

In this concluding chapter, we look to the future, beyond the context of the current COVID-19 syndemic, exploring *what can be done* to decrease health inequalities as the pandemic wears on, and as we begin to emerge from it.

Trends in health inequalities: before and after COVID-19

The COVID-19 crisis has highlighted the extent of social, economic and health inequalities across societies. Even before the pandemic, health inequalities were increasing.[1] For example, while life expectancy in Europe increased for almost all social groups since 1990, behind this headline 'success story' there is also evidence of rising inequalities in some countries, as gains in life expectancy were smaller among men and women with a lower level of education or living in more deprived areas.[2] For example, in England, the gap in life expectancy for women between the most and least deprived areas grew to 7.1 years by 2015.[3] In Scotland, analysis of data up to 2017 found that deaths under age 65 had actually increased in recent years, reflecting worsening mortality rates among the most socioeconomically disadvantaged populations.[4] In the US, there was a marked increase in the all-cause mortality of middle-aged White non-Hispanic men and women, particularly those in lower income groups, between 1999 and 2013.[5] These increases in health inequalities were partly a result of increases in 'deaths of despair', such as those related to suicide or alcohol and drug use, as well as the impacts of austerity (see Chapter Four).[6]

There is also emerging evidence that inequalities in the health impact of COVID-19 is in turn reducing life expectancy gains with, for example, life expectancy declines of around one year on average in England and Wales between 2019 and 2020 as a result of the syndemic pandemic.[7] These immediate COVID-19 related decreases in life expectancy are likely to be higher in the most deprived areas and among the groups that this book (see Chapter Two) has shown have been most adversely impacted by COVID-19, including lower socioeconomic groups and racial/ethnic minorities. The indirect impact of COVID-19 on health, as a result of the emergency responses (see Chapter Three); deaths from other causes that couldn't be treated because of the COVID-19 focus in healthcare;[8] and the pandemic's economic crisis (see Chapter Four); are also likely to be unequally distributed, with already disadvantaged groups again faring worse. Additionally, for the reasons explored in Chapters Three and Four, there is an unequal impact by gender, with women (on average) having been more impacted by lockdown restrictions (for example, as a result of relatively larger caring roles) and by job losses (given the sectors affected). Once again, all of this seems likely to increase health inequalities into the future.

As this book has shown (notably in Chapter Two), inequalities in COVID-19 deaths have been driven by underlying inequalities in clinical risk factors and chronic conditions such as diabetes, heart disease and other non-communicable diseases (NCDs). These risk factors and NCDs are, in turn, related to the social and commercial determinants of health (see Chapter One), including economic inequalities (see Chapter Four). To reduce these longstanding, underlying health inequalities, and in turn reduce inequalities emerging from any future pandemics (rather than repeating the patterns of the past, as we see happening now, with inequalities in COVID-19 deaths shadowing those of the 1918 pandemic flu), we need to address inequalities in NCDs. This is not an easy task,[9] but there is recent evidence from two case studies (Germany in the 1990s and England in the 2000s) of how this can be done through acting on the social and commercial determinants of health through social and economic policies (see Chapter Five).[10]

Reducing health inequalities case study 1: German reunification in the 1990s[11]

In 1990, the life expectancy gap between the former East and former West Germany was almost three years for women and three and a half years for men. This gap rapidly narrowed in the following decades so that by 2010 it had dwindled to just a few months for women (West: 82.8 years; East: 82.6 years) and just over one year for men (West: 78.0 years, East: 76.6 years).[12] This provides an important case study in how health inequalities can be reduced: significantly, at scale and in a fairly short time frame. How was this done?

Firstly, after the reunification of the former East and West Germany, living standards of East Germans improved with increases in wage levels and better access to a variety of foods and consumer goods.[13] This particularly benefitted old age pensioners in the East, as the West German pension system was extended into the East, resulting in very large increases in income for older East Germans.[14] Research by scholars at the Max Planck Institute for Demographic Research in Rostock has shown that the rapid improvement in life expectancy in 1990s East Germany was largely a result of falling death rates among pensioners.[15]

Secondly, immediately after reunification, considerable financial support was given to modernise the hospitals and healthcare equipment in the East, and the availability of nursing care, screening and pharmaceuticals also increased. This raised standards of healthcare in the East so that they were comparable to those of the West within just a few years.[16] This had notable impacts on, for example, neonatal mortality and mortality from conditions amenable to prevention (for example, cancer screening) or medical treatment.[17,18]

Both the improvement in living standards and the increased investment in healthcare were the result of the deep and sustained *political* decision to reunify Germany as fully as possible so that 'what belongs together will grow together'.[19] Indeed, the improvements in the East were funded by a special Solidarity Surcharge: an additional income tax charge paid across Germany.[20]

Reducing health inequalities case study 2: English health inequalities strategy in the 2000s

In 1997, a Labour government was elected in the UK on a manifesto that included a commitment to reducing health inequalities. This led to the implementation, between 1998 and 2010, of a wide-ranging and multifaceted health inequalities reduction strategy for England, in which policymakers systematically and explicitly attempted to reduce inequalities in health. The strategy focused specifically on: supporting families; engaging communities in tackling deprivation; improving prevention; increasing access to healthcare; and tackling the underlying social determinants of health. For example, the strategy included large increases in levels of public spending on a range of social programmes; the introduction of the national minimum wage; area-based interventions such as the Health Action Zones; and a substantial increase in expenditure on the healthcare system. Alongside this, the UK also implemented a series of changes designed to tackle a key commercial determinant of health via a series of legislation to reduce tobacco marketing and promotion and, separately, to reduce people's exposure to secondhand smoke. These efforts collectively led to the UK leading an international comparison of tobacco control measures in 2010.[21] What was the impact of these efforts on health inequalities?

Collectively, these policies led to reductions in social inequalities in the key social determinants of health, including unemployment, child poverty, housing quality, access to healthcare and educational attainment.[22] This was accompanied by modest reductions in health inequalities between the most deprived areas in England and the rest of the country: inequalities in life expectancy decreased by just over a year for men and around six months for women;[23] the gap in infant mortality rates narrowed by 12 infant deaths per 100,000 births per year; and inequalities in mortality amendable to healthcare interventions decreased by 35 deaths per 100,000 for men and 16 deaths per 100,000 for women.[24] The impact of tobacco control measures on health inequalities is less clear, partly because this has been under-researched, though average levels of tobacco consumption did decline throughout this period.[25] Complicating matters, the legislative interventions described (which changed people's social and environmental context by restricting their exposure to tobacco marketing and secondhand smoke) were increasingly accompanied by policy efforts to encourage individual behaviour change; precisely the kinds of intervention now recognised as increasing inequalities.[26]

So, the English strategy of the 2000s reduced health inequalities, but the decreases were on the modest side. Arguably, it may have been even more effective if there had not been a gradual 'lifestyle drift' in governance, whereby policy often shifted from acknowledging the impact of social determinants of health to focusing on individual-level behaviour change when it came to policies and interventions.[27] Crucially, the strategy did not explicitly attempt to address economic inequality, focusing on the less ambitious task of addressing poverty, and therefore did not seek to address more fundamental social and economic causes of inequality.[28] While some policies focused on these fundamental causes, there was, however, little substantial redistribution of income across society. The strategy might also have been even more effective had it been sustained over a longer time period.

The German and English case studies show that it is possible to reduce health inequalities by improving social and economic conditions. We need to learn from these past experiences, and quickly, to prevent inequality growing post-COVID-19 and to reduce health inequalities in the future. We can act to create a more equitable future by changing both what our governments do (our policies) and how our governments respond to, and engage with, their citizens (our politics).

Lessons for a post-COVID-19 future: policy

To contain the COVID-19 pandemic and minimise its effects in the short term, we need social policies that allow workers, particularly those who have been deemed essential workers, to protect themselves and their families as well as the members of the public with whom they might come into contact. Paid time off work in case of illness is another essential tool to combat the spread of COVID-19, but in some countries (for example, the US) and for some workers (for example, self-employed, informal sector workers) sickness leave is not a right. It should be.

Universal access to healthcare that is affordable and of a high quality is clearly also needed so that people do not defer care, including a possible COVID-19 diagnosis, due to cost or to a lack of healthcare providers in their area. Societies in which there are high financial, cultural or geographic barriers to accessing healthcare must make breaking down these barriers a priority.

In societies where the spread of the virus has not been contained, it may be necessary to close all but essential businesses and services, leading to massive loss of employment and income. Unemployment insurance benefits and short-work arrangements must be expanded to cover sectors of the economy that have until now not been covered (for example, gig and contract workers, informal sector workers, some self-employed). Meanwhile, essential workers must be guaranteed as a matter of right the safest possible working conditions, adequate PPE at no cost, full sickness pay in the event that they contract COVID-19, and care services for children and elders as needed.

Other immediate policy actions that can help prevent the growth of further inequalities in the midst of the COVID-19 pandemic include cash and nutrition assistance to help those who have lost their jobs survive the effects of lockdown. The latter may seem extreme, with hunger confined to the poorest residents of countries with limited safety nets. But food banks across Europe have reported sizeable increases in demand for food aid (for example, a 40% rise in France) compared to the pre-pandemic period.[29] And the need has grown so great in the UK that in December 2020 the United Nations Children's Fund (UNICEF) provided financing for food assistance to needy children in South London, the first time in the agency's 70-year history that it has provided emergency food aid in Britain. School-based meal programmes and other food entitlements such as the US's SNAP (Supplemental Nutrition Assistance Program) should be maintained or expanded so long as economic crisis leads to hungry families.

Governments must also acknowledge that lockdowns can have highly variable effects on mental and physical health depending on the type of housing and neighbourhoods where people live. Where privacy, greenspace, and grocery outlets are in short supply, governments must allow latitude for residents to travel for exercise and essential food items. Expanded access to mental health services is also urgently needed to help protect against the psychological stresses of both social isolation and economic disruption, which are otherwise likely to increase the burden of mental illness.[30]

If we get the immediate policy response to the COVID-19 pandemic right, we can limit the inequality that might otherwise be created, and also end the pandemic more quickly. This is because many of the policies that reduce inequality in the impact of COVID-19 also reduce the overall incidence of the disease. As case rates in a community drop, the disease will spread more slowly, and vaccination campaigns will have a better chance of halting its spread altogether. Within the next year to 18 months, then, societies that act now to reduce COVID-19 inequalities will likely move beyond the immediate need to contain the spread of infection, and into a phase of recovery. As we move into this next phase, we must focus on policies that can cut through the COVID-19 social inequality syndemic by altering the distribution of upstream social determinants of health.

Access to healthcare and other social protections for people who are already sick will continue to be important as we exit from the pandemic, just as they were before it. But the greatest benefits for health equity will come from introducing or strengthening social policies that act on the social determinants of health. To take just one such social determinant, housing, as an example, governments could act in a variety of ways to ensure access to safe, affordable housing: through reforms to zoning policies to allow for increased housing construction in high-cost areas; through regulations to ease access to mortgage credit for first-time home buyers; through rental subsidies; and/ or through direct government provision of housing. Similarly, more stringent regulation of environmental hazards could help to reduce the burden of disease in communities that are disproportionately exposed to air, water, and noise pollution.[31]

Most critical of all for breaking the syndemic cycle are those social and labour market policies aimed at reducing poverty and inequality, and with them the morbidity and mortality associated with both absolute and relatively low socioeconomic status.[32] A vast array of policies is available to combat poverty, from reforms to the tax system to job guarantees, from living wage ordinances and advanced maintenance (child support) directives to support for labour rights. Any of these policies will help reduce health inequalities, since resource poverty is a key social determinant of health. However, health does not only improve when one goes from being poor to not-poor, but also as one rises up the entire social gradient.[33]

Since most people in the global north (at least 80% of the population in most countries) are not resource-poor, policies that reduce inequality, and not only poverty, have an extremely important role to play in ensuring that our emergence from the pandemic is equitable and healthy.[34] When we reduce inequality, we reduce poverty, but also increase the disposable income of middle-class families. This allows middle-income people to live less-stressed, healthier lives, and relieves the burden on social welfare programmes. Reductions in socioeconomic inequality can be achieved through macroeconomic policies that aim to stimulate investment and job growth; by establishing a living minimum wage and fostering productive bargaining between the social partners; through tax reforms that shift the burden of financing public goods away from those with incomes near the middle of the income distribution and toward those with the highest earnings and wealth (including real estate and other assets); and through more public financing of healthcare and tertiary education expenses that would otherwise be borne out of pocket by middle-class families.

Clearly, a thriving economy is necessary to generate employment, income, and tax revenues, all of which are necessary in order to ensure individual and societal wellbeing. Strong social protection is generally compatible with economic performance, but research has found that certain types of social policies are particularly valuable.[35] Two aspects of social policy, income protection policies and support for families, have particularly important implications for both economic performance and health, and are areas in which many countries could do more to promote health equality.

Times of crisis can also act as windows of opportunity for those seeking to change policy,[36] and it is possible that some governments will respond to the COVID-19-induced economic crisis by pursuing more innovative economic policies. Prior to the pandemic, policymakers in Iceland, New Zealand and Scotland were already collaborating to attempt to achieve a shift away from traditional mechanisms for achieving economic growth, towards a focus on policy approaches such as 'inclusive growth' and 'wellbeing economies', which prioritise social and environmental wellbeing and greater inclusivity. Since the outbreak of COVID-19, these ideas have gained traction, with Wales and Finland both joining the official 'Wellbeing Economies Governments Partnership'.[37]

Significant disruptions to employment and earnings are likely to continue across multiple sectors of the economy even as we begin to recover from the pandemic. Yet unemployment insurance and assistance benefits have been reduced in many OECD countries over the last 20 years.[38] This will leave many workers vulnerable once the immediate relief provisions put in place during the pandemic expire. In order to serve as effective social shock absorbers during the pandemic recovery, unemployment benefits must be adequate to maintain household consumption during prolonged periods of unemployment, and protect all workers, regardless of the sector of the economy or the type of job tenure. Other forms of wage protection, such as the wage insurance or *kurzarbeit* systems (short-time working: a governmental unemployment insurance system in which employees accept a reduction in working time and pay, with the state making up for all or part of the lost wages) used in Germany and Denmark, may be even more valuable during the recovery from COVID-19.[39] Such programmes not only protect workers' ability to support themselves and their families; they also support the economy by allowing employers to rehire workers quickly and without loss of firm-specific skills.[40] Emergency support for small businesses to retain salaried workers during the pandemic has been a welcome relief to many firms and employees, and should be regularised and expanded to support economic recovery.

Support for families with young children will also be needed to promote economic recovery. Most rich democracies also now have leave policies that support fathers in taking time off to care for young children, which encourages mothers' re-employment and fathers' engagement with children, both of which promote longer-terms gains for household earnings and child wellbeing.[41] Affordable, high-quality childcare and early childhood education are also critical for parents' ability to return to work after the birth of a child, as well as for child development and subsequent earning potential.[42,43] Making society work better for parents with young children can help boost the employment and earnings of both non-family paid caregivers and parents, which are necessary for economic recovery in the medium term; this is an important long-term investment in the health and productivity of our future workforce. Societies that already provide a sufficient array of benefits for families with young children should ensure that these policies are prioritised as parents return to work, to avoid prolongation of women's disproportionate exit from the labour force during COVID-19. In countries that currently lack paid parental leave and publicly financed childcare, such as the US, steps must be taken to fill these gaps in order to ensure child wellbeing and the re-entry of women into the workplace.

Strong welfare states also protect our collective health by generating an enhanced sense of social solidarity and trust. Generous public social programmes are associated with higher levels of trust in others and in the government,[44] and some research has shown that this association is the result of robust welfare states causing people to be more trusting.[45] For both individuals and societies, having greater trust in other people is associated with better health outcomes.[46,47] Moreover, we know from previous research that in pandemic situations, individuals are more likely to cooperate with rules issued by trusted leaders.[48] Thus, investing in social welfare systems that promote social cohesion and trust in government is not only good for population health, equity, and economic recovery, but also essential for our survival.

Lessons for a post-COVID-19 future: politics

To prevent the pandemic from creating worse inequalities, we need not only policy change, but also political change: changes to our political parties and institutions that can lead to a greater voice for working people, and limit the outsized and growing influence of elite, corporate and financial sector actors whose short-term interests are promoted by inequality.

Decades of political science research have shown that socioeconomic inequality very often both results from and translates into political inequality: people of lower socioeconomic status participate in politics at lower rates, and are even further underrepresented in politics because of their higher rates of incarceration and death.[49,50] Furthermore, political elites are less responsive to the policy preferences of constituents with lower socioeconomic status than to those of economic elites.[51] Outside of the electoral arena, the preferences of the super-rich and business elites are even more thoroughly reflected in the policymaking of countries like the US and the UK that have followed a decades-long strategy of reducing the influence of working-class people by undermining organised labour.[52,53]

The concentration of resources at the top of the social hierarchy, which (as noted in Chapter Four) has worsened since the outbreak of COVID-19, leads to hoarding behaviour and highly unequal societies.[54] This is because those at the top of the hierarchy seek to protect their social and economic privileges, including the privileges of resuming pre-pandemic patterns of business, consumption, and social life, despite the risks to workers. Until vaccination rates among the entire world population are high enough to ensure herd immunity, the outsized influence of socioeconomic elites in politics is likely to result in continuing waves of the pandemic due to pressure to reopen economies prematurely.

When schools, neighbourhoods, and social worlds are segregated by race/ethnicity and class, it becomes more difficult for the powerful to imagine that they share a common fate with others. Consider, for example, the statement made by a judge of the Supreme Court for the US state of Wisconsin, Justice Patience Roggensack, when his court was asked to consider reversing the Wisconsin Governor's stay-at-home order in May 2020. Roggensack argued that a coronavirus outbreak among meatpacking workers was not grounds for maintaining the lockdown, since it didn't affect 'the regular folks in Brown County'.[55] But we are all in this together, as the people of Wisconsin learned when the virus spread beyond the meatpacking plants to the rest of the state. COVID-19 is not an equal-opportunity killer; but extreme social inequality, for example between poor, immigrant meatpackers and Supreme Court judges, can lead to a failure to recognise our common humanity that ultimately affects all of us.

What kinds of changes to our political life could help remediate the harms done by inequality? To begin with, governments can act to counterbalance the outsized power of economic elites. They can strengthen protections for labour organisation where unions are under threat, and use the power of the state to promote productive dialogue among the social partners. Corporate law can be reformed to encourage accountability through strengthened participation of multiple stakeholders in governance.[56] And antitrust laws can be strengthened to protect competition and prevent very large corporations from amassing even greater power.

Parties form the basis of political competition in democratic systems. Different types of electoral systems (for example, proportional representation versus single-member district systems) are associated with differing levels of attentiveness on the part of political parties to the interests of middle-class, working-class and poor people, and with differing levels of inequality and redistribution.[57,58,59] It is not clear that reforming electoral systems at this point would result in less inequality, but there are things that parties could do on their own to bring about needed change.

First, political parties of the left, centre and right must recognise the harm that has been done by their decades-long accession to neoliberal economic and social policy dogma and associated obsession with ineffective technocratic fixes to inequality. Neither 'activation' policies nor 'investment in human capital' can curb the excessive inequalities generated by unrestrained market forces; but an active programme of regulation and redistribution can be part of a compelling vision for a more equal society.[60] Parties themselves could promote a reorientation of their social and economic policy programmes by undertaking internal reforms that re-prioritise recruitment of people from all walks of life into leadership, rather than drawing from the ranks of elite university graduates and political consultants.

Changing the way that citizens engage in politics can also lead to a greater voice for ordinary people in the policies that shape our lives and our health. Universal civic education, mandatory voting, and time off work for voting and other political activity, could all promote civic engagement by individuals who might otherwise find themselves too busy, or not well enough informed, to participate in politics. Some reforms could even promote direct citizen involvement in policymaking, as we discuss later.

Conclusion: hope in a time of COVID-19

As we look across the rapidly growing scholarly literature that seeks to describe and understand the unfolding consequences of the current syndemic pandemic, we are struck by the consistency with which the crisis is being framed as a moment of significant policy change. In almost every area of major policy concern, authors are arguing that this crisis poses major threats but also offers opportunities for substantive change. This reflects observations that earlier crises have ushered in major policy changes (for example, the creation of welfare states in many European countries following two World Wars), which have sometimes substantially reduced inequalities,[61] leading some to claim that crises have 'paradigm-shattering' qualities.[62] Put simply, ideas previously disregarded as overly radical can suddenly begin to seem less risky in the context of mass upheaval. Change, of course, is not always progressive. However, for those committed to greater equality, there are certainly at least five reasons to be hopeful, as this short section reflects.

First, the pandemic *may stimulate progressive economic reforms.* The immediate economic impacts of the pandemic run largely in the opposite direction, as Chapter Four outlined; a wealthy elite have accumulated shockingly high increases in their personal wealth by betting on the recovery of particular firms; households with high levels of disposable income prior to the pandemic are, in many cases, now wealthier as a result of having less options for spending this money; and many of those in positions of financial precarity have been pushed to the brink and beyond. Yet, not only has COVID-19 shone a bright light on the extent and consequences of economic inequalities, but some governments have also introduced measures that were previously deemed unimaginable, prompting questions about why similar interventions are routinely ruled out in 'normal' times. In the UK (and other countries such as New Zealand and Finland), the Wellbeing Economy Alliance are framing the pandemic as 'an opportunity to transform economies and societies in radically positive directions', noting the lack of popular support for a 'return to the way things were'.[63] Similarly, some have argued that COVID-19 'has exposed the veins of inequality in Latin America and is acting at a critical juncture that could break the silence on issues such as the tax exemptions and privileges enjoyed by the rich'.[64]

Second, in an era that had been labelled 'post-truth', in which 'experts' had been increasingly derided,[65] COVID-19 may have ushered in *a new 'golden age' of scientific expertise*, at least in terms of rejuvenated public and policy credibility and support. In the UK, a government fronted by a senior minister who decried 'the public have had enough of experts' in 2016 had shifted to one repeatedly claiming it is now 'following the science'.[66] Globally, as state-led vaccine rollouts encounter the myths and misinformation propagated by anti-vaccination campaigners,[67] the necessity of combatting 'fake news' is becoming all too clear. While there are dangers in overselling the 'offer' of science and expertise (which provides information that enables societies to make meaningful political choices but does not remove the need for choices to be made), the rejuvenation of scientific expertise and, notably, of public health and epidemiology may afford attention and support to researchers working to improve public health and reduce health inequalities.

Third, while the extent and speed of government responses to COVID-19 are creating pressure points for democracy, providing clear opportunities for a slide towards more authoritarian styles of leadership,[68] this crisis may also be *stimulating democratic rejuvenation*. In many states, COVID-19 has drawn attention to the importance of independent media oversight of government, while also showcasing the flexibility and speed with which civil society can respond to crises.[69] Against this backdrop, policy interest in more participatory forms of governance appears to be increasing. Prior to the pandemic, deliberative democracy was already beginning to take off. Participatory budgeting, an experiment in direct democratic governance pioneered in Porto Alegre, Brazil and later taken up in more than 100 European cities, brought citizens into the policy process by allowing them to express their priorities for public spending.[70] Bigger policy decisions, such as climate change, were being explored via citizens' assemblies, following early experimentation with deliberative forums in Ireland that led to a referendum on same-sex marriage and, later, on removing the longstanding ban on abortions.[71] In the context of the pandemic, the French Convention Citoyenne pour le Climat and the UK Climate Assembly both successfully switched to operating online while, in contrast, many traditional parliaments have struggled.[72] Although these kinds of democratic innovation, which prioritise dialogue rather than opinion change, are certainly no democratic panacea, they do offer means of bringing together publics, experts and decision makers, 'strengthening the science, society, and democracy nexus', rebuilding public engagement and countering some of the unequal power relations inherent within representative democratic systems. Given the role that unequal power relations play in unequal health experiences, efforts to widen and strengthen citizen engagement in policy discussions seem like a welcome development.[73]

Fourth, although the economic crisis may mean policy and public concern with climate change takes a back seat,[74] COVID-19 is also being positioned as *an important learning opportunity for efforts to tackle climate change*.[75] The crisis has demonstrated both the value of scientific expertise and that governments which take decisive preventative action in response to scientific evidence fare far better than those who wait until the disastrous consequences are clear for all to see. Moreover, the improvements in air quality that have followed the massive reductions in travel,[76] combined with the widespread shift to online interactions (for example, for meetings), are providing some hope that it might be possible to reduce vehicle emissions and promote 'active travel' in the longer term.[77] Given the unequal impacts of climate change, and the intricate links between human and planetary health, this too may be good news for those seeking to improve health and reduce inequalities.

Fifth, while some analysts are positing that COVID-19 and associated border closures are accelerating the social exclusion (and, therefore, vulnerability) of migrant and refugee populations, others are arguing that *the pandemic is highlighting the high cost of discrimination*. The COVID-19 pandemic, write Gottlieb and colleagues, 'is a powerful illustration that societies can only be as healthy as their weakest members', providing a strong economic rationale for ensuring healthcare is accessible to all, including migrant and refugee populations.[78] More fundamentally, Sabatello and colleagues argue that, occurring against the backdrop of the Black Lives Matter movement in the US, the pandemic 'gives a face to decades of segregation, racism and structural discrimination [and] forces us to look to the generations of [minority ethnic groups] that have often endured mistreatment in all aspects of life'.[79] Yet again, we find evidence of hope that, in revealing such profound inequities, COVID-19 might serve as a stimulus for greater awareness which, in turn, might translate into sustained social action and, ultimately, meaningful social change.[80]

The syndemic nature of this pandemic is, it seems, both a tragedy and a moment that is inspiring hope 'for repair and a better equitable and sustainable future'.[81] Writing from a South African perspective, Struwig and colleagues posit that 'COVID-19 might constitute the basis for a positive societal transformation that will have a lasting positive influence on our core values, and serve as a catalyst for a social compact that will promote unity to fight against poverty and inequality'.[82] Focusing on children and young people in Australia, Jones and colleagues argue that the 'pandemic can be conceptualised as an opportunity to create a more equitable society'.[83] Reflecting on a multitude of vulnerable populations in the UK, Bhaskar and colleagues argue that COVID-19 makes it 'onerous that systemic issues be addressed and efforts to build inclusive and sustainable societies be pursued to ensure the provision of universal healthcare and justice for all'.[84] Writing from Germany and focusing on the sustainability of cities, Haase argues that the coronavirus crisis can be used as 'an opportunity to re-think and re-discuss the type of sustainability we want to see in our cities'.[85] A WHO report on COVID-19 and health inequalities commented that 'recovery and transition from COVID-19 also provides an unprecedented opportunity to create healthier and more resilient people, societies and economies'.[86]

Almost everywhere we look, we find not only researchers, but also journalists, policymakers, and members of the public making the case that now is the time for a decisive shift towards more equitable policies and social justice. Can we also be hopeful from a health inequalities perspective? Hoping, of course, is insufficient: we must act; but hope allows people to believe that a better future is possible. And this is a first step.

Notes

Preface

[1]   Sydenstricker, 2006 [1931]

Chapter 1

[1]   https://www.lexico.com/en/definition/perfect_storm
[2]   For example, on 23 March 2020 the UK Prime Minister announced that people can only go outside to buy food, to exercise once a day, or to go to work if they absolutely cannot work from home. Citizens will face police fines for failure to comply with these new measures.
[3]   Whitehead, 2007
[4]   Marmot, 2006
[5]   Marmot, 2006
[6]   Bambra, 2016
[7]   London Health Observatory, 2012
[8]   Reid, 2011
[9]   ONS, 2019
[10] ONS, 2019
[11] Schrecker and Bambra, 2015
[12] Marmot, 2010
[13] Robinson et al, 2019
[14] Bambra (ed), 2019
[15] Eikemo et al, 2017
[16] Forster et al, 2018
[17] Roberts, 2011
[18] Berchick et al, 2018
[19] National Center for Health Statistics, 2018
[20] Centers for Disease Control and Prevention, 2018
[21] Centers for Disease Control and Prevention, 2018

22   Jones, 2006
23   Hill, 2015
24   Kapilashrami et al, 2015
25   Hill, 2015
26   Kapilashrami et al, 2015
27   For a more extensive overview of the social determinants of health see Bambra, 2016.
28   Marmot, 2010
29   WHO, 2008
30   Center for American Progress, 2017
31   Greer et al, 2021
32   Thirlway, 2020
33   Collin and Hill, 2015
34   Naa Oyo et al, 2009
35   Macdonald et al, 2018
36   Nguyen et al, 2020
37   Bambra et al, 2020a
38   Singer, 2009
39   Singer, 2000
40   Bambra et al, 2020a
41   Goldblatt et al, 2020

Chapter 2

1   Sydenstricker, 2006 [1931]
2   Lawrence, 2006
3   SkyNews, 27 March 2020
4   Baena-Díez et al, 2020
5   Chen and Krieger, 2020
6   CBC, 2020
7   Sapey et al, 2020
8   ICNARC, 2020
9   de Lusignan et al, 2020
10   Public Health England, 2020
11   Mahase, 2020b
12   Chen and Krieger, 2020
13   Calderon-Larranaga, et al, 2020
14   ONS, 2020a
15   ONS, 2020b
16   National Records of Scotland, 2020
17   Bambra et al, 2020b
18   Ricardo Martins-Filho et al, 2020
19   Olmos and Stuardo, 2020

[20] Arijit Das et al, 2021

[21] ONS, 2020c

[22] National Records of Scotland, 2020

[23] ONS, 2020c

[24] Chen et al, 2021

[25] Chen et al, 2021

[26] Dragano et al, 2020

[27] Estimated relative risks compared to professional occupations ranged from 1.4 to 4.8; see Baral et al, 2021.

[28] Iyengar and Jain, 2020

[29] Biggs et al, 2020

[30] Menachemi et al, 2020

[31] Chen and Krieger, 2020

[32] CBC, 2020

[33] CBC, 2020

[34] CBC, 2020

[35] PHE, 2020

[36] Steyn et al, 2020

[37] Chicago Department of Public Health, 2020

[38] Chen and Krieger, 2020

[39] Bixler, 2020

[40] Egede and Walker, 2020

[41] Qureshi et al, 2020

[42] Gravlee, 2020

[43] Feldman and Bassett, 2020

[44] Gravlee, 2020

[45] Rutter et al, 2012

[46] Rutter et al, 2012

[47] Lowcock et al, 2012

[48] Biggerstaff et al, 2014

[49] Tam et al, 2014

[50] Crighton et al, 2007

[51] Johnson and Mueller, 2002

[52] CDC, 2019

[53] Mamelund, 2006

[54] Grantz et al, 2016

[55] McCracken and Curson, 2003

[56] Bengtsson et al, 2018

[57] Bengtsson et al, 2018

[58] Chowell et al, 2008

[59] Almond, 2006

[60] Rice and Bryder, 2005

[61] Summers et al, 2014

[62] Registrar-General, 1920

[63] Registrar-General, 1920, p24

[64] Johnson, 2006

[65] Mamelund, 1998

[66] Johnson, 2006, p95

[67] Gill, 1928, p276

[68] Hamer, 1918, p8

[69] Johnson, 2006, p101

[70] Pearce et al, 2011

[71] Section adapted from Bambra et al, 2020a.

[72] Singer, 2009

[73] Singer, 2000, p13

[74] Roncon et al, 2020

[75] Alqahtani et al, 2020

[76] Simonnet et al, 2020

[77] Guo et al, 2019

[78] European Commission, 2014

[79] WHO, 2008

[80] Dahlgren and Whitehead, 1991

[81] Bambra, 2011a

[82] Todd et al, 2015

[83] Lacobucci, 2019

[84] Bambra, 2016

[85] Gibson et al, 2011

[86] Clair and Hughes, 2019

[87] McNamara et al, 2017

[88] Bambra, 2016

[89] Rutter et al, 2012

[90] Segerstrom and Miller, 2004

[91] Bartley, 2016

[92] Bambra, 2011b

[93] Whitehead et al, 2016

[94] Biondi et al, 1997

[95] Gkiouleka et al, 2018

[96] Bambra et al, 2020c

Chapter 3

[1] Martinez et al, 2020

[2] Martinez et al, 2020

[3] Walsh et al, 2020

[4] Jordan et al, 2020

[5] Gardner et al, 2020

[6] Himmelstein and Woolhandler, 2020

[7] Barber et al, 2017

[8] Czeisler et al, 2020

[9] Fersia et al, 2020

[10] Gallo et al, 2020

[11] Zadnik et al, 2020

[12] Macpherson et al, 2020, p1

[13] Allen et al, 2017

[14] McNamara et al, 2017

[15] Eikemo et al, 2017

[16] Gardner et al, 2020

[17] O'Connor et al, 2020

[18] Pierce et al, 2020

[19] Pierce et al, 2020

[20] O'Connor et al, 2020

[21] Jacques-Aviñó et al, 2020

[22] Qiu et al, 2020

[23] Pierce et al, 2020

[24] Jacques-Aviñó et al, 2020

[25] Qiu et al, 2020

[26] Stroebe et al, 2007

[27] Keyes et al, 2014

[28] Qiu et al, 2020

[29] Miconi et al, 2021

[30] Miconi et al, 2021

[31] Proto et al, 2021

[32] Furlong and Finnie, 2020

[33] Mathias et al, 2020

[34] Purtle, 2020

[35] Mathias et al, 2020, p7

[36] Reny and Barreto, 2020

[37] He et al, 2020

[38] Pellegrini et al, 2020

[39] Sidor and Rzymski, 2020

[40] Niedzwiedz et al, 2020

[41] Joossens and Raw, 2011

[42] Sidor and Rzymski, 2020

[43] Sidor and Rzymski, 2020

[44] Egbe and Ngobese, 2020

[45] Ryan et al, 2020

[46] Parry and Dewing, 2006

[47] Matzopoulos et al, 2020

[48] Kilian et al, 2021

[49] Kilian et al, 2021

[50] Matzopoulos et al, 2020

[51] Kilian et al, 2021

[52] Miranda, 2011

[53] United Nations, 2020a

[54] Czymara et al, 2020

[55] Manzo and Minello, 2020

[56] Manzo and Minello, 2020, p121

[57] Roesch et al, 2020

[58] Women's Aid, 2020

[59] Zhang, 2020

[60] Mahase, 2020

[61] Mittal and Singh, 2020

[62] Usher et al, 2020

[63] Baig et al, 2020

[64] Boserup et al, 2020

[65] Women's Aid, 2020

[66] Women's Aid, 2020

[67] Women's Aid, 2020

[68] Women's Aid, 2020 p10

[69] Women's Aid, 2020

[70] Yakubovich et al, 2018

[71] Thomas et al, 2020

[72] Wong et al, 2020

[73] Caron et al, 2020

[74] Swedo et al, 2020

[75] Abrams and Dettlaff, 2020, p303

[76] Abrams and Dettlaff, 2020, p303

[77] Education Endowment Foundation, 2020

[78] Neidhoefer et al, 2021, p4

[79] Pensiero et al, 2020

[80] Kim and Asbury, 2020

[81] Kim and Asbury, 2020, p1073

[82] Kim and Asbury, 2020, p1073

[83] De Groot and Lemanski, 2020, p10

[84] Kenway and Holden, 2020

[85] Kenway and Holden, 2020

[86] Ahmad et al, 2020

[87] Smith and Anderson, 2018

[88] Venter et al, 2020

[89] Ugolini et al, 2020

[90] Soga et al, 2020

[91] Shoari et al, 2020

92 Crooks et al, 2020
93 Slater et al, 2020
94 van Tilburg et al, 2020
95 Berg-Weger and Morley, 2020
96 Martins Van Jaarsveld, 2020
97 Luchetti et al, 2020
98 Loades et al, 2020
99 Orben et al, 2020
100 Bu et al, 2020
101 McQuaid et al, 2021
102 Azubuike et al, 2020
103 Eruchalu et al, 2021
104 Eyre et al, 2020
105 Wright, 2021
106 Wright, 2021, p2
107 Wood et al, 2021
108 Wood et al, 2021
109 Wood et al, 2021
110 Wood et al, 2021, p6
111 Peretti-Watel et al, 2021
112 Pleyers, 2020
113 Pleyers, 2020

Chapter 4

1 Bambra et al, 2020a
2 Bambra et al, 2020a
3 Guardian, 2020
4 Global Data, 2020
5 Global Data, 2020
6 Johnson, 2006
7 Bambra, 2016
8 Pew Research Center, 2020
9 UBS, 2020
10 NHSA, 2020
11 Communities in Control, 2020
12 Henry-Parkes, 2020
13 Kim and Asbury 2020, p1073
14 Kim and Asbury 2020, p1073
15 Teachout and Zipfel, 2020
16 Teachout and Zipfel, 2020
17 United Nations, 2020b
18 Amadasun, 2020, p3

[19] Sections of this chapter are adapted from Bambra (ed, chapter 1), 2019, reproduced with permission of Policy Press.

[20] Freeman et al, 2020

[21] Gamble, 2009

[22] Bambra, 2011a

[23] Gerdtham and Ruhm, 2006

[24] Tapia Granados, 2005

[25] Adams, 1981

[26] Ruhm, 2000

[27] Katikireddi et al, 2012

[28] Gili et al, 2013

[29] Economou et al, 2011

[30] Houdmont et al, 2012

[31] Barnes et al, 2017

[32] Vizard and Obolenskaya, 2015

[33] Barr et al, 2012

[34] Corcoran et al, 2015

[35] Zavras et al, 2013

[36] Montgomery et al, 1999

[37] Bambra, 2011b

[38] Montgomery, 1999

[39] Brenner, 1995

[40] Bartley et al, 2006

[41] Bambra and Eikemo, 2009

[42] Bambra et al, 2016

[43] Kondo et al, 2008

[44] Hawton et al, 2016

[45] Valkonen et al, 2000

[46] Manderbacka et al, 2001

[47] Dahl and Elstad 2000

[48] Lundberg et al, 2001

[49] Lahlema et al, 2002

[50] Lahelma et al, 2002

[51] Bambra et al, 2013

[52] Petersen et al, 2009

[53] Burstrom et al, 2010

[54] Channing et al, 2020

[55] Bambra et al, 2013

[56] Lahlema et al, 2002

[57] Eikemo and Bambra, 2008

[58] Bambra and Eikemo, 2009

[59] Eikemo and Bambra, 2008

[60] Beckfield et al, 2015

[61] Navarro et al, 2006
[62] Chung and Muntaner, 2006
[63] Popham et al, 2013
[64] Chung and Muntaner, 2006
[65] Lundberg et al, 2008
[66] Beckfield and Bambra, 2015
[67] Abrams and Dettlaff, 2020
[68] Abrams and Dettlaff, 2020
[69] Gamble, 2009
[70] Bambra (ed), 2019
[71] Karanikolos and Kentikelenis, 2016
[72] Karanikolos and Kentikelenis, 2016
[73] Akhter et al, 2018
[74] Akhter et al, 2018
[75] Beatty and Fothergill, 2014
[76] Beatty and Fothergill, 2014
[77] Beatty and Fothergill, 2014
[78] Browne and Levell, 2010
[79] Green et al, 2017
[80] Taylor-Robinson et al, 2019
[81] Hirsch and Stone, 2020
[82] There are approximately 1300 McDonald's restaurants in the UK, according to the company but there are at least 2000 food banks in the UK: FullFact, 2019.
[83] Bambra et al, 2020c
[84] Marmot et al, 2020
[85] Knight et al, 2018, p190
[86] OECD, 2015
[87] McLaughlin and Rank, 2018
[88] Hirsch, 2008
[89] Marmot et al, 2020
[90] Stuckler and Basu, 2013
[91] Karanikolos et al, 2013
[92] Stuckler et al, 2009
[93] Dorling, 2018
[94] Grootegoed and Smith, 2018
[95] Tyler, 2020
[96] Mattheys et al, 2018, p1282
[97] Barr et al, 2015
[98] ONS, 2015
[99] Moeller, 2013
[100] MacLeavy, 2011
[101] Niedzwiedz et al, 2016

[102] Walker et al, 2013, p221
[103] Walker et al, 2013, p221
[104] Walker et al, 2013, p221
[105] Krieger et al, 2008
[106] A political and economic approach favouring free-market capitalism, deregulation, and low government spending.
[107] Schrecker and Bambra, 2015
[108] Blakely et al, 2008
[109] Pearce et al, 2006
[110] Scott-Samuel et al, 2014
[111] Walkerdine, 2010, p111
[112] Smith and Anderson, 2018
[113] Garnham, 2015, p325

Chapter 5

[1] Taleb, 2010
[2] Sequoia Capital, 2020
[3] Bezirtzoglou et al, 2011
[4] Patz et al, 1996
[5] Wu et al, 2016
[6] Wucker, 2016
[7] Hopkin et al, 2016
[8] In reality the complexity of modern systems of social protection means that there are many more than three 'types', depending on the countries, time periods, policies and attributes one includes (see Ferrera, 1996; Walker and Wong, 2005; Bambra, 2007).
[9] Esping-Andersen, 1990
[10] Wilkinson and Pickett, 2009
[11] Scruggs and Allan, 2006
[12] MacDonald and Shildrick, 2013
[13] Cooper and Lu, 2018
[14] Sigurdsson et al, 2020
[15] Kirkevold et al, 2020
[16] Nyashanu et al, 2020, p3
[17] Nyashanu et al, 2020, p3
[18] Sylvers, 2021
[19] Karaca-Mandic et al, 2020
[20] Gilardino, 2020
[21] Gilardino, 2020
[22] Iacobucci, 2020
[23] Bonalumi et al, 2020
[24] BMJ, 2020

25 Augustin et al, 2020
26 Collins et al, 2019
27 Bambra, 2005
28 WHO, 2008
29 Pierson, 2011
30 Pierson, 2011
31 Hopkin and Lynch, 2016
32 Lynch, 2020
33 O'Reilly, 2020
34 O'Reilly, 2020, p10
35 Gershon 2020
36 Bambra et al, 2020d
37 Fortin, 2020
38 Tyler, 2020
39 Pierson, 2000
40 Esping-Andersen, 1990
41 Lynch, 2020
42 Kavaliunas et al, 2020
43 OECD, 2020
44 EUROMOMO, 2020
45 Public Health Agency of Sweden, 2020
46 Lynch, 2014
47 Castles, 2010
48 Bremmer, 2020
49 Kennelly, 2020
50 Lindeman, 2021

Chapter 6

1   Forster et al, 2018
2   Mackenbach et al, 2016
3   Department of Health and Social Care, 2017
4   Walsh et al, 2020
5   Case and Deaton, 2015
6   Case and Deaton, 2020
7   Aburto et al, 2020
8   Hanna et al, 2020
9   Lynch, 2020
10 Bambra, 2016
11 Adapted from Bambra, 2016
12 Kibele et al, 2015
13 Parkes, 1997
14 Gjonça et al, 2000

[15] Gjonça et al, 2000

[16] Nolte et al, 2002

[17] Nolte et al, 2002

[18] Nolte et al, 2000

[19] Bambra, 2016

[20] Gokhale et al, 1994

[21] Joossens and Raw, 2011

[22] Barr et al, 2017

[23] Barr et al, 2017

[24] Barr et al, 2014

[25] ONS, 2016

[26] Lorenc et al, 2013

[27] Whitehead and Popay, 2010

[28] Lynch, 2020

[29] FEBA, 2020

[30] Pfefferbaum and North, 2020

[31] See for example Marmot, 2010

[32] Wilkinson and Pickett, 2009

[33] Marmot, 2010

[34] Marmot, 2010

[35] Atkinson, 2015

[36] Boin et al, 2008

[37] See Wellbeing Economy Alliance https://wellbeingeconomy.org/new wego-member-finland

[38] Scruggs and Allan, 2006

[39] https://www.bloomberg.com/news/articles/2020-04-03/how-germany-pays-workers-when-their-work-dries-up-quicktake

[40] Thelen, 2014

[41] Morris et al, 2019

[42] Morrissey, 2009

[43] Heckman et al, 2010

[44] Cammett et al, 2015

[45] Brewer et al, 2014

[46] Barefoot et al, 1998

[47] Giordano et al, 2012

[48] Prati et al, 2011

[49] Cottrell et al, 2019

[50] Jacobs and Skocpol, 2005

[51] Gilens, 2012

[52] Hacker and Pierson, 2010

[53] Hopkin and Shaw, 2016

[54] Reeves, 2017

[55] https://www.washingtonpost.com/nation/2020/05/07/meatpacking-workers-wisconsin-coronavirus/

[56] Palladino and Karlsson, 2018

[57] Iversen and Soskice, 2006

[58] Jusko, 2017

[59] Anderson and Beramendi, 2012

[60] Lynch, 2020

[61] Scheidel, 2017

[62] Boin et al, 2008

[63] See Wellbeing Economy Alliance https://wellbeingeconomy.org/new-wego-member-finland

[64] Cimini et al, 2020

[65] Brown, 2016

[66] Pérez-González, 2020

[67] Hajela, 2020

[68] Parry et al, 2020

[69] Thomas and Whitehead, 2020

[70] Sintomer et al, 2008

[71] Palese, 2018

[72] Cousins, 2020

[73] McCartney et al, 2021

[74] Ecker et al, 2020

[75] Klenert et al, 2020

[76] Rodríguez-Urrego and Rodríguez-Urrego, 2020

[77] Nurse and Dunning, 2020

[78] Gottlieb et al, 2020

[79] Sabatello et al, 2020

[80] Krieger, 2020

[81] Krieger, 2020

[82] Struwig et al, 20020

[83] Jones et al, 2020

[84] Bhaskar et al, 2020

[85] Haase, 2020

[86] Goldblatt et al, 2020, p13

References

Abrams, L. and Dettlaff, A. (2020) Voices from the frontlines: social workers confront the COVID-19 pandemic, *Social Work*, 65: 302–5.

Aburto, J., Kashyap, R., Schöley, J., Angus, C., Ermisch, J., Mills, M. and Beam Dowd, J. (2020) Estimating the burden of COVID-19 pandemic on mortality, life expectancy and lifespan inequality in England and Wales: a population-level analysis, *medRxiv*, doi: https://doi.org/10.1101/2020.07.16.20155077

Adams, O. (1981) *Health and Economic Activity: A Time-Series Analysis of Canadian Mortality and Unemployment Rates 1950–1977*, Ottawa: Minister of Supply and Services Canada.

Ahmad, K., Erqou, S., Shah, N., Nazir, U., Morrison, A.R., Choudhary, G. and Wu, W-C. (2020) Association of poor housing conditions with COVID-19 incidence and mortality across US counties, *PLOS ONE*, 15(11): e0241327.

Akhter, N., Bambra, C., Mattheys, K., Warren, J. and Kasim, A. (2018) Inequalities in mental health and well-being in a time of austerity: longitudinal findings from the Stockton-on-Tees cohort study, *SSM – Population Health*, 6: 75–84, https://doi.org/10.1016/j.ssmph.2018.08.004

Allen, L., Williams, J., Townsend, N., Mikkelsen, B., Roberts, N., Foster, C. and Wickramasinghe, K. (2017) Socioeconomic status and non-communicable disease behavioural risk factors in low-income and lower-middle-income countries: a systematic review, *The Lancet Global Health*, 5(3): e277–e289.

Almond, D. (2006) Is the 1918 influenza pandemic over? Long-term effects of in utero influenza exposure in the post-1940 US population, *Journal of Political Economy*, 114: 672–712.

Alqahtani, J., Oyelade, T., Aldhahir, A.M., Alghamdi, S.M., Almemahdi, M., Alqahtani, A.S., Quaderi, S., Mandal, S. and Hurst, J.R. (2020) Prevalence, severity and mortality associated with COPD and smoking in patients with COVID-19: a rapid systematic review and meta-analysis, *PLOS ONE*, 15(5): e0233147.

Amadasun, S. (2020) From coronavirus to 'hunger virus': mapping the urgency of social work response amid COVID-19 pandemic in Africa, *International Social Work*, doi:10.1177/0020872820959366

Anderson, C.J. and Beramendi, P. (2012) Left parties, poor voters, and electoral participation in advanced industrial societies, *Comparative Political Studies*, 45(6): 714–46.

Arijit Das, S., Kalikinkar, D., Tirthankar, B., Ipsita D. and Manob, D. (2021) Living environment matters: unravelling the spatial clustering of COVID-19 hotspots in Kolkata megacity, India, *Sustainable Cities and Society*, 65: 102577.

Atkinson, A.B. (2015) *Inequality: What Can Be Done?* Cambridge, MA: Harvard University Press.

Augustin, M., Schommers, P., Suárez, I., Koehler, P., Gruell, H., Klein, F., Maurer, C., Langerbeins, P., Priesner, V., Schmidt-Hellerau, K. and Malin, J.J. (2020) Rapid response infrastructure for pandemic preparedness in a tertiary care hospital: lessons learned from the COVID-19 outbreak in Cologne, Germany, February to March 2020, *Eurosurveillance*, 25(21): 2000531, doi:10.2807/1560-7917.ES.2020.25.21.2000531

Azubuike, O.B., Adegboye, O. and Quadri, H. (2020) Who gets to learn in a pandemic? Exploring the digital divide in remote learning during the COVID-19 pandemic in Nigeria, *International Journal of Educational Research Open*, https://doi.org/10.1016/j.ijedro.2020.100022

Baena-Díez, J.M., Barroso, M., Cordeiro-Coelho, S.I., Díaz, J.L. and Grau, M. (2020) Impact of COVID-19 outbreak by income: hitting hardest the most deprived, *Journal of Public Health*, https://www.ncbi.nlm.nih.gov/pmc/articles/PMC7454748/

Baig, M.A.M., Ali, S. and Tunio, N.A. (2020) Domestic violence amid COVID-19 pandemic: Pakistan's perspective, *Asia Pacific Journal of Public Health*, 32(8): 525–6.

Bambra, C. (2005) Cash versus services: 'worlds of welfare' and the decommodification of cash benefits and healthcare services, *Journal of Social Policy*, 34(2): 195–213.

Bambra, C. (2007) Going beyond the three worlds of welfare capitalism: regime theory and public health research, *Journal of Epidemiology and Community Health*, 61: 1098–102.

Bambra, C. (2011a) *Work, Worklessness and the Political Economy of Health*, Oxford: Oxford University Press.

Bambra, C. (2011b) Work, worklessness and the political economy of health inequalities, *Journal of Epidemiology and Community Health*, 65: 746–50.

Bambra, C. (2016) *Health Divides: Where You Live Can Kill You*, Bristol: Policy Press.

Bambra, C. (ed) (2019) *Health in Hard Times: Austerity and Health Inequalities*, Bristol: Policy Press.

Bambra, C. and Eikemo, T. (2009) Welfare state regimes, unemployment and health: a comparative study of the relationship between unemployment and self-reported health in 23 European countries, *Journal of Epidemiology and Community Health*, 63: 92–8.

Bambra, C., Copeland, A., Nylen, C., Curtis, S., Kasim, A. and Burstrom, B. (2013) All in it together? Recessions, health and health inequalities in England and Sweden, 1991 to 2010, American Geographical Association Annual Conference, Los Angeles, CA.

Bambra, C., Garthwaite, K., Copeland, A. and Barr, B. (2016) All in it together? Health inequalities, welfare austerity and the 'Great Recession', in K.E. Smith, S. Hill and C. Bambra (eds) *Health Inequalities: Critical Perspectives*, Oxford: Oxford University Press, pp 164–76.

Bambra, C., Riordan, R., Ford, J. and Matthews, F. (2020a) The COVID-19 pandemic and health inequalities, *Journal of Epidemiology and Community Health*, https://jech.bmj.com/content/early/2020/06/13/jech-2020-214401

Bambra, C., Munford, L., Alexandros, A., Barr, B., Brown, H., Davies, H., Konstantinos, D., Mason, K., Pickett, K., Taylor, C., Taylor-Robinson, D. and Wickham, S. (2020b) *COVID-19 and the northern powerhouse: tackling inequalities for UK health and productivity*, Newcastle: NHSA, https://www.thenhsa.co.uk/app/uploads/2020/11/NP-COVID-REPORT-101120-.pdf

Bambra, C., Norman, P. and Johnson, N. (2020c) Visualising regional inequalities in the 1918 Spanish flu pandemic in England and Wales, *Environment and Planning A: Space and Economy*, https://doi.org/10.1177/0308518X20969420

Bambra, C., Albani, V. and Franklin, P. (2020d) COVID-19 and the gender health paradox, *Scandinavian Journal of Public Health*, https://doi.org/10.1177/1403494820975604

Baral, S., Chandler, R., Prieto, R., Gupta, S., Mishra, S. and Kulldorff, M. (2021) Leveraging epidemiological principles to evaluate Sweden's COVID-19 response, *Annals of Epidemiology*, 54: 21–6.

Barber, R.M., Fullman, N., Sorensen, R.J., Bollyky, T., McKee, M., Nolte, E., Abajobir, A.A., Abate, K.H., Abbafati, C., Abbas, K.M. and Abd-Allah, F. (2017) Healthcare access and quality index based on mortality from causes amenable to personal healthcare in 195 countries and territories, 1990–2015: a novel analysis from the Global Burden of Disease Study 2015, *The Lancet*, 390(10091): 231–66.

Barefoot, J.C., Maynard, K.E., Beckham, J.C., Brummett, B.H., Hooker, K. and Siegler, I.C. (1998) Trust, health, and longevity, *Journal of Behavioral Medicine*, 21(6): 517–26.

Barnes, M.C., Donovan, J.L., Wilson, C., Chatwin, J., Davies, R., Potokar, J., Kapur, N., Hawton, K., O'Connor, R. and Gunnell, D. (2017) Seeking help in times of economic hardship: access, experiences of services and unmet need, *BMC Psychiatry*, 17: 84.

Barr, B., Taylor-Robinson, D., Scott-Samuel, A., McKee, M. and Stuckler, D. (2012) Suicides associated with the 2008–10 economic recession in England: time trend analysis, *BMJ*, 345, doi: https://doi.org/10.1136/bmj.e5142

Barr, B., Bambra, C. and Whitehead, M. (2014) The impact of NHS resource allocation policy on health inequalities in England 2001–11: longitudinal ecological study, *BMJ*, 348, doi: https://doi.org/10.1136/bmj.g3231

Barr, B., Kinderman, P. and Whitehead, M. (2015) Trends in mental health inequalities in England during a period of recession, austerity and welfare reform 2004–2013, *Social Science and Medicine*, 147: 324–31.

Barr, B., Higgerson, J. and Whitehead, M. (2017) Investigating the impact of the English health inequalities strategy: time trend analysis, *BMJ*, 26: 358, doi:https://doi.org/10.1136/bmj.j3310

Bartley, M., Ferrie, J. and Montgomery, S.M. (2006) Health and labour market disadvantage: unemployment, non-employment, and job insecurity, in M. Marmot and R.G. Wilkinson (eds), *Social Determinants of Health*, Oxford: Oxford University Press, pp 78–96.

Bartley, M. (2016) *Health Inequality: An Introduction to Concepts, Theories and Methods*, 2nd edn, Cambridge: Polity Press.

Beatty, C. and Fothergill, S. (2014) The local and regional impact of the UK's welfare reforms, *Cambridge Journal of Regions Economy and Society*, 7(1): 63–79.

Beckfield, J. and Bambra, C. (2015) Shorter lives, stingier states: welfare shortcomings help explain the US mortality disadvantage, *Social Science and Medicine*, 170: 30–8.

Beckfield, J., Bambra, C., Eikemo, TA., Huijts, T. and Wendt, C. (2015) Towards an institutional theory of welfare state effects on the distribution of population health, *Social Theory and Health*, 13, 227–44.

Bengtsson, T., Dribe, M. and Eriksson, B. (2018) Social class and excess mortality in Sweden during the 1918 influenza pandemic, *American Journal of Epidemiology*, 187: 2568–76.

Berchick, E., Hood, E. and Barnett, J. (2018) *Health insurance coverage in the United States: 2017*, Washington DC: US Census Bureau, https://www.census.gov/library/publications/2018/demo/p60-264.html

Berg-Weger, M., Morley, J.E. (2020) Loneliness and social isolation in older adults during the COVID-19 pandemic: implications for gerontological social work, *Journal of Nutrition, Health and Ageing*, 24(5): 456–8.

Bezirtzoglou, C., Dekas, K., Charvalos, E. (2011) Climate changes, environment and infection: facts, scenarios and growing awareness from the public health community within Europe, *Anaerobe*, 17(6): 337–40, doi:10.1016/j.anaerobe.2011.05.016

Bhaskar, S., Rastogi, A., Menon, K.V., Kunheri, B., Balakrishnan, S. and Howick, J. (2020) Call for action to address equity and justice divide during COVID-19, *Frontiers in Psychiatry*, 11:1411.

Biggerstaff, M., Jhung, M.A., Reed, C., Garg, S., Balluz, L., Fry, A.M. and Finelli, L. (2014) Impact of medical and behavioural factors on influenza-like illness, healthcare-seeking, and antiviral treatment during the 2009 H1N1 pandemic: United States, 2009–2010, *Epidemiology and Infection*, 142: 114–25.

Biggs, H.M., Harris, J.B., Breakwell, L., Dahlgren, F.S., Abedi, G.R., Szablewski, C.M., Drobeniuc, J., Bustamante, N.D., Almendares, O., Schnall, A.H. and Gilani, Z. (2020) Estimated community seroprevalence of SARS-CoV-2 antibodies: two Georgia counties, April 28–May 3, 2020, *Morbidity and Mortality Weekly Report*, 69: 965–70, doi: http://dx.doi.org/10.15585/mmwr.mm6929e2

Biondi, M. and Zannino, L.G. (1997) Psychological stress, neuroimmunomodulation, and susceptibility to infectious diseases in animals and man: a review, *Psychotherapy and Psychosomatics*, 66: 3–26.

Bixler, D. (2020) SARS-CoV-2: associated deaths among persons aged <21 years: United States, February 12–July 31, 2020, *Morbidity and Mortality Weekly Report*, doi: http://dx.doi.org/10.15585/mmwr.mm6937e4external icon

Blakely, T., Tobias, M. and Atkinson, J. (2008) Inequalities in mortality during and after restructuring of the New Zealand economy: repeated cohort studies, *BMJ*, 336(7640): 371–5.

BMJ (2020) On the front lines of the response to COVID-19 in Spain: a nation under a state of emergency, https://blogs.bmj.com/bmj/2020/03/31/on-the-front-lines-of-the-response-to-covid-19-in-spain-a-nation-under-a-state-of-emergency/ (Accessed 12 January 2021)

Boin, A., McConnell, A. and Hart, P. (2008) *Governing After Crisis: The Politics of Investigation, Accountability and Learning*, Cambridge: Cambridge University Press.

Bonalumi, G., di Mauro, M., Garatti, A., Barili, F., Gerosa, G. and Parolari, A. (2020) The COVID-19 outbreak and its impact on hospitals in Italy: the model of cardiac surgery, *European Journal of Cardio-Thoracic Surgery*, 57(6): 1025–28, doi:10.1093/ejcts/ezaa151

Boserup, B., McKenney, M. and Elkbuli, A. (2020) Alarming trends in US domestic violence during the COVID-19 pandemic, *American Journal of Emergency Medicine*, 38(12): 2753–5.

Bremmer, I. (2020) The best global responses to the COVID-19 pandemic, *Time*, 12 June 2020, https://time.com/5851633/best-global-responses-covid-19/ (Accessed 26 January 2021)

Brenner, H. (1995) Political economy and health, in B. Amick, S. Levine, A.R. Tarlov and D.C. Walsh (eds), *Society and Health*, Oxford: Oxford University Press, pp 211–46.

Brewer, K.B., Oh, H. and Sharma, S. (2014) 'Crowding in' or 'crowding out'? An examination of the impact of the welfare state on generalized social trust, *International Journal of Social Welfare*, 23(1): 61–8.

Brown, T. (2016) Evidence, expertise, and facts in a 'post-truth' society, *BMJ*, 355: i6467.

Browne, J. and Levell, P. (2010) *The Distributional Effect of Tax and Benefit Reforms to Be Introduced between June 2010 and April 2014: A Revised Assessment*, London: Institute for Fiscal Studies.

Bu, F., Steptoe, A. and Fancourt, D. (2020) Who is lonely in lockdown? Cross-cohort analyses of predictors of loneliness before and during the COVID-19 pandemic, *Public Health*, 186: 31–4.

Burstrom, B., Whitehead, M., Clayton, S., Fritzell, S., Vannoni, F. and Costa, G. (2010) Health inequalities between lone and couple mothers and policy under different welfare regimes: the example of Italy, Sweden and Britain, *Social Science and Medicine*, 70(6): 912–20.

Calderon-Larranaga, A., Vetrano, D.L., Rizzuto, D., Bellander, T., Fratiglioni, L. and Dekhtyar, S. (2020) High excess mortality during the COVID-19 outbreak in Stockholm region areas with young and socially vulnerable populations, *BMJ Global Health*, 5: e003595, doi:10.1136/bmjgh-2020-003595

Cammett, M., Lynch, J. and Bilev, G. (2015) The influence of private health care financing on citizen trust in government, *Perspectives on Politics*, 938–57.

Caron, F., Plancq, M C., Tourneux, P., Gouron, R. and Klein, C. (2020) Was child abuse underdetected during the COVID-19 lockdown? *Archives de Pédiatrie: Organe Officiel de la Société Francaise de Pédiatrie*, 27(7): 399–400, https://doi.org/10.1016/j.arcped.2020.07.010

Case, A. and Deaton, A. (2015) Rising midlife morbidity and mortality: US Whites, *Proceedings of the National Academy of Sciences*, 112(49):15078–83.

Case, A. and Deaton, A. (2020) *Deaths of Despair and the Future of Capitalism*, Princeton, NJ: Princeton University Press.

Castles, F.G. (2010) The English-speaking countries, in F.G. Castles, S. Leibfried, J. Lewis, H. Obinger and C. Pierson (eds), *The Oxford Handbook of the Welfare State*, 1st edn, Oxford: Oxford University Press, doi:10.1093/oxfordhb/9780199579396.003.0043

CBC (Canadian Broadcasting Company) (2020) Lower income people, new immigrants at higher COVID-19 risk in Toronto, data suggests, https://www.cbc.ca/news/canada/toronto/low-income-immigrants-covid-19-infection-1.5566384 (Accessed 4 July 2020)

CDC (Centers for Disease Control and Prevention) (2018) Health of Black or African American non-Hispanic population, https://www.cdc.gov/nchs/fastats/black-health.htm

CDC (2019) 1918 Pandemic (H1N1 virus), https://www.cdc.gov/flu/pandemic-resources/1918-pandemic-h1n1.html

Center for American Progress (2017) Health disparities by race and ethnicity, https://www.americanprogress.org/issues/race/reports/2020/05/07/484742/health-disparities-race-ethnicity/#:~:text=In%202017%2C%2010.6%20percent%20of,health%20insurance%20coverage%20in%202017

Channing, A., Davies, R., Gabriel, S., Harris, L., Makrelov, K., Robinson, S., Levy, S., Simbanegavi, W., van Seventer, D. and Anderson, L. (2020) COVID-19 lockdowns, income distribution, and food security: an analysis for South Africa, *Global Food Security*, 26: 1000410.

Chen, J.T. and Krieger, N. (2020) Revealing the unequal burden of COVID-19 by income, race/ethnicity, and household crowding: US county vs ZIP code analyses, Harvard Center for Population and Development Studies Working Paper Series, 19(1), https://tinyurl.com/ya44we2r

Chen, Y., Glymour, M., Riley, A., Balmes, J., Duchowny, K., Harrison, R., Matthay, E. and Bibbins-Domingo, K. (2021) Excess mortality associated with the COVID-19 pandemic among Californians 18–65 years of age, by occupational sector and occupation, *medRxiv* 2021.01.21.21250266, doi: https://doi.org/10.1101/2021.01.21.21250266

Chicago Department of Public Health (2020) COVID-19 death characteristics for Chicago residents, https://www.chicago.gov/city/en/sites/covid-19/home/latest-data.html (Accessed 5 July 2020)

Chowell, G., Bettencourt, L.M.A., Johnson, N., Alonso, W.J. and Viboud, C. (2008) The 1918–1919 influenza pandemic in England and Wales: spatial patterns in transmissibility and mortality impact, *Proceedings of the Royal Society B: Biological Sciences*, 275: 501–9.

Chung, H. and Muntaner, C. (2006) Political and welfare state determinants of infant and child health indicators: an analysis of wealthy countries, *Social Science & Medicine*, 63(3): 829–42.

Cimini, F., Julião, N., de Souza, A. and Cabral, N. (2020) COVID-19 pandemic, social mitigation and taxation: the open veins of inequality in Latin America, *Bulletin of Latin American Research*, 39: 56–61.

Clair, A. and Hughes, A. (2019) Housing and health: new evidence using biomarker data, *Journal of Epidemiology and Community Health*, 73(3): 256.

Collin, J. and Hill, S. (2015) Industrial epidemics and inequalities: the commercial sector as a structural driver of inequalities in non-communicable diseases, in K.E. Smith, C. Bambra and S.E. Hill (eds) *Health Inequalities: Critical Perspectives*, Oxford: Oxford University Press, pp 177–91.

Collins, S.R., Bhupal, H.K. and Doty, M.M. (2019) Health insurance coverage eight years after the ACA: fewer uninsured Americans and shorter coverage gaps, but more underinsured, Commonwealth Fund, https://doi.org/10.26099/penv-q932

Communities in Control (2020) Leading the COVID recovery, https://locality.org.uk/policy-campaigns/leading-the-coronavirus-recovery/ (Accessed 4 November 2020)

Cooper, C.L. and Lu, L. (eds) (2018) *Presenteeism at Work*, Cambridge: Cambridge University Press.

Corcoran, P., Griffin, E., Arensman, E., Fitzgerald, A.P. and Perry, I.J. (2015) Impact of the economic recession and subsequent austerity on suicide and self-harm in Ireland: an interrupted time series analysis, *International Journal of Epidemiology*, 44: 969–77.

Cottrell, D., Herron, M.C., Rodriguez, J.M. and Smith, D.A. (2019) Mortality, incarceration, and African American disenfranchisement in the contemporary United States, *American Politics Research*, 47(2): 195–237.

Cousins, C. (2020) How parliaments are working during the COVID-19 pandemic, Oireachtas Library & Research Service, https://data.oireachtas.ie/ie/oireachtas/libraryResearch/2020/2020-05-01_1-rs-note-how-parliaments-are-working-during-the-covid-19-pandemic_en.pdf

Crighton, E.J., Elliott, S.J., Moineddin, R., Kanaroglou, P. and Upshur, R. (2007) A spatial analysis of the determinants of pneumonia and influenza hospitalizations in Ontario (1992–2001), *Social Science and Medicine,* 64: 1636–50.

Crooks, K., Casey, D. and Ward, J.S. (2020) First Nations people leading the way in COVID-19 pandemic planning, response and management, *Medical Journal of Australia*, 213(4): 151–2.

Czeisler, M.É., Marynak, K., Clarke, K.E., Salah, Z., Shakya, I., Thierry, J.M., Ali, N., McMillan, H., Wiley, J.F., Weaver, M.D. and Czeisler, C.A. (2020) Delay or avoidance of medical care because of COVID-19-related concerns: United States, *Morbidity and Mortality Weekly Report*, 69(36): 1250–7.

Czymara, C.S., Langenkamp, A. and Cano, T. (2020) Cause for concerns: gender inequality in experiencing the COVID-19 lockdown in Germany, *European Societies*, 1–14, doi:10.1080/14616696.2020.1808692

Dahl, E., and Elstad, J.I. (2000) Recent changes in social structure and health inequalities in Norway, *Scandinavian Journal of Public Health*, 55 (Suppl): 7–17.

Dahlgren, G. and Whitehead, M. (1991) *Policies and Strategies to Promote Social Equity in Health*, Stockholm: Institute for Future Studies.

De Groot, J. and Lemanski, C. (2020) COVID-19 responses: infrastructure inequality and privileged capacity to transform everyday life in South Africa, *Environment and Urbanization*, https://doi.org/10.1177/0956247820970094

de Lusignan, S., Dorward, J., Correa, A., Jones, N., Akinyemi, O., Amirthalingam, G., Andrews, N., Byford, R., Dabrera, G., Elliot, A. and Ellis, J. (2020) Risk factors for SARS-CoV-2 among patients in the Oxford Royal College of General Practitioners Research and Surveillance Centre primary care network: a cross-sectional study, *The Lancet Infectious Diseases*, doi:https://doi.org/10.1016/S1473-3099(20)30371-6

Department of Health and Social Care (2017) *Annual Report and Accounts 2016–17*, London: DHSC.

Dickinson, E. (1891) *Poems by Emily Dickinson*, 2nd series, Boston, MA: Little, Brown.

Dorling, D. (2018) Rise in mortality in England and Wales in first seven weeks of 2018, *BMJ*, 360: k1090.

Dragano, N., Rupprecht, C.J., Dortmann, O., Scheider, M. and Wahrendorf, M. (2020) Higher risk of COVID-19 hospitalization for unemployed: an analysis of 1,298,416 health insured individuals in Germany, doi: https://doi.org/10.1101/2020.06.17.20133918

Ecker, U., Butler, L., Cook, J., Hurlstone, M., Kurz, T. and Lewandowsky, S. (2020) Using the COVID-19 economic crisis to frame climate change as a secondary issue reduces mitigation support, *Journal of Environmental Psychology*, 70: 101464.

Economou, M., Madianos, M., Theleritis, C., Peppou, L. and Stefanis C. (2011) Increased suicidality amid economic crisis in Greece, *The Lancet*, 378: 1459.

Education Endowment Foundation (2020) Impact of school closures on the attainment gap: Rapid Evidence Assessment, https://educationendowmentfoundation.org.uk/public/files/EEF_(2020)_-_Impact_of_School_Closures_on_the_Attainment_Gap.pdf: Education Endowment Foundation

Egbe, C.O. and Ngobese, S.P. (2020) COVID-19 lockdown and the tobacco product ban in South Africa, *Journal of Tobacco Induced Diseases,* doi: 10.18332/tid/120938

Egede, L. and Walker, R. (2020) Structural racism, social risk factors, and COVID-19: a dangerous convergence for Black Americans, *New England Journal of Medicine*, 383: e77.

Eikemo, T.A. and Bambra, C. (2008) The welfare state: a glossary for public health, *Journal of Epidemiology and Community Health*, 62: 3–6.

Eikemo, T.A., Bambra, C., Huijts, T. and Fitzgerald, R. (2017) The European Social Survey (ESS) rotating module on the social determinants of health: the first pan-European sociological health inequalities survey, *European Sociological Review*, 3: 137–53.

Eruchalu, C.N., Pichardo, M.S., Bharadwaj, M., Rodriguez, C.B., Rodriguez, J.A., Bergmark, R.W., Bates, D.W. and Ortega, G. (2021) The expanding digital divide: digital health access inequities during the COVID-19 pandemic in New York City, *Journal of Urban Health*, doi: 10.1007/s11524-020-00508-9

Esping-Andersen, G. (1990) *The Three Worlds of Welfare Capitalism*, Princeton, NJ: Princeton University Press.

EUROMOMO (2020) EuroMOMO Bulletin, Week 53, https://euromomo.eu/dev-404-page/ (Accessed 12 January 2021)

European Commission (2014) *Roma health report: Health status of the Roma population in the member states of the European Union,* Brussels: European Commission, https://ec.europa.eu/health/sites/health/files/social_determinants/docs/2014_roma_health_report_en.pdf (Accessed 22 April 2020)

Eyre, D.W., Lumley, S.F., O'Donnell, D., Campbell, M., Sims, E., Lawson, E., Warren, F., James, T., Cox, S., Howarth, A. and Doherty, G. (2020) Differential occupational risks to healthcare workers from SARS-CoV-2: A prospective observational study: doi: 10.7554/eLife.60675

FEBA (2020) *European Food Banks in a Post COVID-19 Europe,* FEBA Report, 1, European Food Banks Federation, July 2020, https://lp.eurofoodbank.org/wp-content/uploads/2020/07/FEBA_Report_Survey_COVID_July2020.pdf

Feldman, J. and Bassett, M. (2020) The relationship between neighborhood poverty and COVID-19 mortality within racial/ethnic groups (Cook County, Illinois), doi: https://doi.org/10.1101/2020.10.04.20206318

Ferrera, M. (1996) The 'southern model' of welfare in social Europe, *Journal of European Social Policy,* 6(1): 17–37.

Fersia, O., Bryant, S., Nicholson, R., McMeeken, K., Brown, C., Donaldson, B., Jardine, A., Grierson, V., Whalen, V. and Mackay, A. (2020) The impact of the COVID-19 pandemic on cardiology services, doi: 10.1136/openhrt-2020-001359

Forster, T., Kentikelenis, A. and Bambra, C. (2018) Health inequalities in Europe: setting the stage for progressive policy action, Foundation for European Progressive Studies and Action on Social Change (TASC), https://www.feps-europe.eu/component/attachments/attachments.html?task=attachment&id=168

Fortin, J. (2020) After meat workers die of COVID-19, families fight for compensation, *The New York Times,* 6 October, https://www.nytimes.com/2020/10/06/business/coronavirus-meatpacking-plants-compensation.html (Accessed 19 November 2020)

Freeman, T., Gesesew, H., Bambra, C., Regina, E., Popay, J., Sanders, D., Macinko, J., Musolino, C. and Baum, F. (2020) Why do some countries do better or worse in life expectancy relative to wealth: an analysis of three countries: Brazil, Ethiopia, and the US, *International Journal for Equity in Health*, 19: 202.

FullFact (2019) Are there more foodbanks than McDonalds in the UK? http://fullfact.org/electionlive/2019/dec/9/food-banks-more-mcdonalds/

Furlong, Y. and Finnie, T. (2020) Culture counts: the diverse effects of culture and society on mental health amidst COVID-19 outbreak in Australia, *Irish Journal of Psychological Medicine*, 37(3): 237–42.

Gallo, O., Locatello, L.G., Orlando, P., Martelli, F., Bruno, C., Cilona, M., Fancello, G., Mani, R., Vitali, D., Bianco, G. and Trovati, M. (2020) The clinical consequences of the COVID-19 lockdown: a report from an Italian referral ENT department, Laryngoscope *Investigative Otolaryngology*, 5(5): 824–31.

Gamble, A., (2009) *The Spectre at the Feast: Capitalist Crisis and the Politics of Recession*, Basingstoke: Palgrave.

Gardner, T., Fraser, C. and Peytrignet, S. (2020) Elective care in England: assessing the impact of COVID-19 and where next, The Health Foundation, https://www.health.org.uk/publications/long-reads/elective-care-in-england-assessing-the-impact-of-covid-19-and-where-next

Garnham, L. (2015) Understanding the impacts of industrial change and area-based deprivation on health inequalities, using Swidler's concepts of cultured capacities and strategies of action, *Social Theory and Health*, 13(3–4): 308–39

Gerdtham, U. and Ruhm, C. (2006) Deaths rise in good economic times: evidence from the OECD, *Economics and Human Biology*, 4: 298–316.

Gershon, L. (2020) COVID-19's impact on working women is an unprecedented disaster, *Smithsonian Magazine*, https://www.smithsonianmag.com/smart-news/covid-19s-impact-working-women-unprecedented-disaster-180976084/ (Accessed 8 December 2020)

Gibson, M., Petticrew, M., Bambra, C., Sowden, A.J., Wright, K.E. and Whitehead, M. (2011) Housing and health inequalities: a synthesis of systematic reviews of interventions aimed at different pathways linking housing and health, *Health and Place*, 17: 175–84.

Gilardino, R.E. (2020) Does 'flattening the curve' affect critical care services delivery for COVID-19? A global health perspective, *International Journal of Health Policy and Management*, doi:10.34172/ijhpm.2020.117

Gilens, M. (2012) *Affluence and Influence: Economic Inequality and Political Power in America*, Princeton: Princeton University Press.

Gili, M., Roca, M., Basu, S., McKee, M. and Stuckler, D. (2013) The mental health risks of economic crisis in Spain: evidence from primary care centres, 2006 and 2010, *European Journal of Public Health*, 23(1): 103–8.

Gill, C.A. (1928) *The Genesis of Epidemics and the Natural History of Disease*, London: Bailliere, Tindall and Cox.

Giordano, G.N., Björk, J. and Lindström, M. (2012) Social capital and self-rated health: a study of temporal (causal) relationships, *Social Science & Medicine*, 75(2): 340–8.

Gjonça, A., Brockmann, H. and Maier, H. (2000) Old-age mortality in Germany prior to and after reunification, *Demographic Research*, 3, http://www.jstor.org/stable/26348006

Gkiouleka, A., Huijts, T., Beckfield, J. and Bambra, C. (2018) Understanding the micro and macro politics of health: inequalities, intersectionality and institutions: a research agenda, *Social Science and Medicine*, 200: 92–8.

Global Data (2020) COVID-19 Executive Briefing Report, https://www.globaldata.com/covid-19/ (Accessed 4 November 2020)

Gokhale, J., Raffelhuschen, B. and Walliser, J. (1994) The burden of German unification: a generational accounting approach, *Working Papers (Old Series)*, Federal Reserve Bank of Cleveland, pp 141–65, RePEc:fip:fedcwp:9412

Goldblatt, P., Shriwise, A., Yang, L. and Brown, C. (2020) Health inequity and the effects of COVID-19: assessing, responding to and mitigating the socioeconomic impact on health to build a better future, WHO Europe, https://apps.who.int/iris/bitstream/handle/10665/338199/WHO-EURO-2020-1744-41495-56594-eng.pdf

Gottlieb, N., Trummer, U., Davidovitch, N., Krasnik, A., Juárez, S.P., Rostila, M., Biddle, L. and Bozorgmehr, K. (2020) Economic arguments in migrant health policymaking: proposing a research agenda, *Global Health*, 16: 113, https://doi.org/10.1186/s12992-020-00642-8

Grantz, K.H., Rane, M.S., Salje, H., Glass, G.E., Schachterle, S.E. and Cummings, D.A.T. (2016) Disparities in influenza mortality and transmission related to sociodemographic factors within Chicago in the pandemic of 1918, *Proceedings of the National Academy of Sciences*, 113(48): 13839–44, doi: 10.1073/pnas.1612838113

Gravlee, C. (2020) Systemic racism, chronic health inequities, and COVID-19: a syndemic in the making?, *American Journal of Human Biology*, 32(5): e23482, doi:10.1002/ajhb.23482

Green, J.M., Buckner, S., Milton, S., Powell, K., Salway, S. and Moffatt, S. (2017) A model of how targeted and universal welfare entitlements impact on material, psycho-social and structural determinants of health in older adults, *Social Science & Medicine*, 187: 20–8.

Greer, S., Lynch, J., Reeves, A., Kalousova, L., Gingrich, J., Cylus, J. and Bambra, C. (forthcoming, 2021) *The Politics of Healthy Ageing: Crisis, Controversy, Coalitions*, Cambridge: Cambridge University Press.

Grootegoed, E. and Smith, M. (2018) The emotional labour of austerity: how social workers reflect and work on their feelings towards reducing support to needy children and families, *British Journal of Social Work*, 48: 1929–47.

Guardian (2020) The Great Frost, https://www.theguardian.com/business/2020/nov/25/deadly-frost-and-war-with-the-french-britains-recession-of-the-1700s (Accessed 4 November 2020)

Guo, L., Wei, D., Zhang, X., Wu, Y., Li, Q., Zhou, M. and Qu, J. (2019) Clinical features predicting mortality risk in patients with viral pneumonia: the MuLBSTA score, *Frontiers in Microbiology*, 10: 2752, doi:10.3389/fmicb.2019.02752

Haase, A. (2020) COVID-19 as a social crisis and justice challenge for cities, *Frontiers in Sociology*, 5: 93.

Hacker, J.S. and Pierson, P. (2010) Winner-take-all politics: public policy, political organization, and the precipitous rise of top incomes in the United States, *Politics & Society*, 38(2): 152–204.

Hajela, R. (2020) Public health agencies must burst the vaccine misinformation bubble on social media, LSE Blog, https://blogs.lse.ac.uk/medialse/2020/11/09/public-health-agencies-must-burst-the-vaccine-misinformation-bubble-on-social-media/

Hamer, W. (1918) *Report of the County Medical Officer of Health and School Medical Officer for the Year 1918*, London: London County Council.

Hanna, T., Aggarwal, A., Booth, C. and Sullivan, R. (2020) Counting the invisible costs of COVID-19: the cancer pandemic, *BMJ*, https://blogs.bmj.com/bmj/2020/11/05/counting-the-invisible-costs-of-covid-19-the-cancer-pandemic/

Hawton, K., Bergen, H. and Geulayov, G. (2016) Impact of the recent recession on self-harm: a longitudinal ecologic and patient level investigation from multicentre study of self-harm in England, *Journal of Affective Disorders*, 191, doi:10.1016/j.jad.2015.11.001

He, M., Xian, Y., Lv, X., He, J. and Ren, Y. (2020) Changes in body weight, physical activity, and lifestyle during the semi-lockdown period after the outbreak of COVID-19 in China: an online survey, *Disaster Medicine and Public Health Preparedness*, 1–6, doi: 10.1017/dmp.2020.237

Heckman, J.J., Moon, S.H., Pinto, R., Savelyev, P.A. and Yavitz, A. (2010) The rate of return to the HighScope Perry Preschool Program, *Journal of Public Economics*, 94(1–2): 114–28.

Henry-Parkes, C.M. (2020) Estimating poverty impacts of coronavirus: microstimulation estimates, *Institute for Public Policy Research*, https://www.ippr.org/research/publications/estimating-poverty-impacts-of-coronavirus

Hill, S. (2015) Axes of health inequalities and intersectionality, in K.E. Smith and C. Bambra (eds) *Health Inequalities: Critical Perspectives*, Oxford: Oxford University Press.

Himmelstein, D.U. and Woolhandler, S. (2020) The US healthcare system on the eve of the COVID-19 epidemic: a summary of recent evidence on its impaired performance, *International Journal of Health Services*, 50(4): 408–14.

Hirsch, D. (2008) *Estimating the costs of child poverty*, York: Joseph Rowntree Foundation, https://www.jrf.org.uk/sites/default/files/jrf/migrated/files/2313.pdf

Hirsch, D. and Stone, J. (2020) *Local Indicators of Child Poverty after Housing Costs, 2018/19: Summary of Estimates of Child Poverty after Housing Costs in Local Authorities and Parliamentary Constituencies, 2014/15 – 2018/19*, Loughborough: Loughborough University, https://www.lboro.ac.uk/media-centre/press-releases/2020/october/child-poverty-rise-shapest-in-midlands-and-north/

Hopkin, J. and Lynch, J. (2016) Winner-take all politics in Europe? European inequality in comparative perspective, *Politics and Society*, 44(3): 335–43.

Hopkin, J. and Shaw, K.A. (2016) Organized combat or structural advantage? The politics of inequality and the winner-take-all economy in the United Kingdom, *Politics & Society*, 44(3): 345–71.

Houdmont, J., Kerr, R. and Addley, K. (2012) Psychosocial factors and economic recession: the Stormont Study, *Occupational Medicine*, 62(2): 98–104.

Iacobucci, G. (2020) COVID-19: all non-urgent elective surgery is suspended for at least three months in England, *BMJ*, 368: m1106 doi:10.1136/bmj.m1106

ICNARC (Intensive Care National Audit and Research Centre) (2020) *ICNARC report on COVID-19 in critical care 12 June 2020*, London: Intensive Care National Audit and Research Centre.

Iversen, T. and Soskice, D. (2006) Electoral institutions and the politics of coalitions: why some democracies redistribute more than others, *American Political Science Review*, 165–81.

Iyengar, K.P. and Jain, V.K. (2020) COVID-19 and the plight of migrants in India, *Postgraduate Medical Journal*, doi: 10.1136/postgradmedj-2020-138454

Jacobs, L.R. and Skocpol, T. (eds) (2005) *Inequality and American Democracy: What We Know and What We Need to Learn*, New York: Russell Sage Foundation.

Jacques-Aviñó, C., López-Jiménez, T., Medina-Perucha, L., de Bont, J., Gonçalves, A.Q., Duarte-Salles, T. and Berenguera, A. (2020) Gender-based approach on the social impact and mental health in Spain during COVID-19 lockdown: a cross-sectional study, *BMJ Open*, 10(11): e044617.

Johnson, N. (2001) 1918–1919 influenza pandemic mortality in England and Wales, Data Collection, UK Data Service, SN: 4350, http://doi.org/10.5255/UKDA-SN-4350-1

Johnson, N. (2006) *Britain and the 1918–19 Influenza Pandemic: A Dark Epilogue*, London: Routledge.

Johnson, N. and Mueller, J. (2002) Updating the accounts: global mortality of the 1918–1920 'Spanish' influenza pandemic, *Bulletin of the History of Medecine*, 76(1): 105–15, doi: 10.1353/bhm.2002.0022

Jones, B., Woolfenden, S., Pengilly, S., Breen, C., Cohn, R., Biviano, L., Johns, A., Worth, A., Lamb, R., Lingam, R. and Silove, N. (2020) COVID-19 pandemic: the impact on vulnerable children and young people in Australia, *Journal of Paediatric Child Health*, 56(12): 1851–5, doi: 10.1111/jpc.15169

Jones, D.S. (2006) The persistence of American Indian health disparites, *American Journal of Public Health*, 96(12): 2122–34.

Joossens, L. and Raw, M. (2011) The Tobacco Control Scale 2010 in Europe, *Association of European Cancer Leagues*, https://www.tobaccocontrolscale.org/TCS2010.pdf

Jordan, R.E., Adab, P. and Cheng, K.K. (2020) COVID-19: risk factors for severe disease and death, *BMJ*, 368: m1198.

Jusko, K.L. (2017) *Who Speaks for the Poor? Electoral Geography, Party Entry, and Representation*, Cambridge: Cambridge University Press.

Juvenal (100 AD) Satires V1, 165 https://www.gutenberg.org/files/50657/50657-h/50657-h.htm

Kapilashrami, A., Hill, S. and Meer, N. (2015) What can health inequalities researchers learn from an intersectionality perspective? Understanding social dynamics with an inter-categorical approach?, *Social Theory and Health*, 13: 288–307.

Karaca-Mandic, P., Sen, S., Georgiou, A., Zhu, Y. and Basu, A. (2020) Association of COVID-19-related hospital use and overall COVID-19 mortality in the US, *Journal of General Internal Medicine*, 1–3, doi:10.1007/s11606-020-06084-7

Karanikolos, M. and Kentikelenis, A. (2016) Health inequalities after austerity in Greece, *International Journal for Equity in Health*, 15: 83.

Karanikolos, M., Mladovsky, P., Cylus, J., Thomson, S., Basu, S., Stuckler, D., Mackenbach, J.P. and McKee, M. (2013) Financial crisis, austerity, and health in Europe, *The Lancet*, 381(9874): 1323–31.

Katikireddi, S.V., Niedzwiedz, C.L. and Popham, F. (2012) Trends in population mental health before and after the 2008 recession: a repeat cross-sectional analysis of the 1991–2010 Health Surveys of England, *BMJ Open*, 2(5), doi: 10.1136/bmjopen-2012-001790

Kavaliunas, A., Ocaya, P., Mumper, J., Lindfeldt, I. and Kyhlstedt, M. (2020) Swedish policy analysis for COVID-19, *Health Policy and Technology*, 9(4): 598-612, doi:10.1016/j.hlpt.2020.08.009

Kennelly, B., O'Callaghan, M. and Coughlan, D. (2020) The COVID-19 pandemic in Ireland: an overview of the health service and economic policy response, *Health Policy and Technology*, 9(4): 419–29, doi:10.1016/j.hlpt.2020.08.021

Kenway, P. and Holden, J. (2020) *Accounting for the Variation in the Confirmed COVID-19 Caseload across England: An Analysis of the Role of Multi-generation Households, London and Time*. London: New Policy Institute.

Keyes, K., Pratt C., Galea, S., McLaughlin, K.A, Koenen, K.C. and Shear, K. (2014) The burden of loss: unexpected death of a loved one and psychiatric disorders across the life course in a national study, *American Journal of Psychiatry*, 171(8): 864–71.

Kibele, E.U.B., Kluesener, S. and Scholz, R. (2015) Regional mortality disparities in Germany: long-term dynamics and possible determinants, *Kolner Zeitschrift Fur Soziologie Und Sozialpsychologie*, 67: 241–70.

Kilian, C., Rehm, J., Allebeck, P., Braddick, F., Gual, A., Barták, M., Bloomfield, K., Gil, A., Neufeld, M., O'Donnell, A. and Petruželka, B. (2021) Alcohol consumption during the COVID-19 pandemic in Europe: a large-scale cross-sectional study in 21 countries, *Research Square*, https://www.researchsquare.com/article/rs-148341/v2

Kim, L.E. and Asbury, K. (2020) 'Like a rug had been pulled from under you': the impact of COVID-19 on teachers in England during the first six weeks of the UK lockdown, *British Journal of Educational Psychology*, 90: 1062–83.

Kirkevold, Ø., Eriksen, S., Lichtwarck, B. and Selbæk, G. (2020) Smittevern på sykehjem under COVID-19-pandemien, *Sykepl Forsk,* 15: e-81554, doi:10.4220/Sykepleienf.2020.81554

Klenert, D., Funke, F., Mattauch, L. and O'Callaghan, B. (2020) Five lessons from COVID-19 for advancing climate change mitigation, *Environmental and Resource Economics*, 76: 751–78, https://doi.org/10.1007/s10640-020-00453-w

Knight, A., O'Connell, R. and Brannen, J. (2018) Eating with friends, family or not at all: young people's experiences of food poverty in the UK, *The Children's Society*, 32: 185–94.

Kondo, N., Subramanian, S., Kawachi, I., Takeda, Y. and Yamagata, Z. (2008) Economic recession and health inequalities in Japan: analysis with a national sample, 1986–2001, *Journal of Epidemiology and Community Health*, 62: 869–75.

Krieger, N. (2020) ENOUGH: COVID-19, structural racism, police brutality, plutocracy, climate change-and time for health justice, democratic governance, and an equitable, sustainable future, *American Journal of Public Health*, 110(11):1620–3, doi:10.2105/AJPH.2020.305886

Krieger, N., Rehkopf, D.H., Chen, J.T., Waterman, P.D., Marcelli, E. and Kennedy, M. (2008) The fall and rise of US inequities in premature mortality: 1960–2002, *PLOS Medicine*, 5(2): 227–41.

Lacobucci, G. (2019) GPs in deprived areas face severest pressures, *BMJ*, 365: l2104.

Lahelma, E., Kivelä, K., Roos, E., Tuominen, T., Dahl, E., Diderichsen, F., Elstad, J.I., Lissau, I., Lundberg, O., Rahkonen, O. and Rasmussen, N.K. (2002) Analysing changes of health inequalities in the Nordic welfare states, *Social Science and Medicine*, 55(4): 609–25.

Lawrence, A.J. (2006) The incidence of influenza among persons of different economic status during the epidemic of 1918 (1931): commentary, *Public Health Reports*, 121(Suppl 1): 190.

Lindeman, T. (2020) What Canada's COVID response can teach the US about social safety nets, *Fortune*, https://fortune.com/2020/10/23/canada-unemployment-cerb-economy-growth-coronavirus/ (Accessed 26 January 2021)

Loades, M.E, Chatburn, E., Higson-Sweeney, N., Reynolds, S., Shafran, R., Brigden, A., Linney, C., McManus, M.N., Borwick, C. and Crawley, E. (2020) Rapid systematic review: the impact of social isolation and loneliness on the mental health of children and adolescents in the context of COVID-19, *Journal of the American Academy of Child & Adolescent Psychiatry*, 59(11): 1218–39.e1213.

London Health Observatory (2012) *Health Inequalities Overview*, London: Public Health England.

Lorenc, T., Petticrew, M., Welch, V. and Tugwell, P. (2013) What types of interventions generate inequalities? Evidence from systematic reviews, *Journal of Epidemiology and Community Health*, 67: 190–3.

Lowcock, E.C., Rosella, L.C., Foisy, J., McGeer, A. and Crowcroft, N. (2012) The social determinants of health and pandemic H1N1 2009 influenza severity, *American Journal of Public Health*, 102: 51–8.

Luchetti, M., Lee, J.H., Aschwanden, D., Sesker, A., Strickhouser, J., Terracciano, A. and Sutin, A. (2020) The trajectory of loneliness in response to COVID-19, *American Psychologist*, 75, 10.1037/amp0000690.

Lundberg, O., Diderichsen, F. and Yngwe, M.Å. (2001) Changing health inequalities in a changing society? Sweden in the mid-1980s and mid-1990s, *Scandinavian Journal of Public Health*, 29: 31–9.

Lundberg, O., Yngwe, M.Å., Stjärne, M.K., Elstad, J.I., Ferrarini, T., Kangas, O., Norström, T., Palme, J. and Fritzell, J. (2008) The role of welfare state principles and generosity in social policy programmes for public health: an international comparative study, *The Lancet*, 372(9650): 1633–40.

Lynch, J.A. (2014) Cross-national perspective on the American welfare state, in D. Beland, K. Morgan and C. Howard (eds) *Oxford Handbook of US Social Policy*, Oxford: Oxford University Press, doi:10.1093/oxfordhb/9780199838509.013.023

Lynch, J. (2020) *Regimes of Inequality: The Political Economy of Health and Wealth*, Cambridge: Cambridge University Press.

Macdonald, L., Olsen, J., Shortt, N. and Ellaway, A. (2018) Do 'environmental bads' such as alcohol, fast food, tobacco, and gambling outlets cluster and co-locate in more deprived areas in Glasgow City, Scotland? *Health & Place*, 51: 224–31.

MacDonald, R. and Shildrick, T. (2013) Youth and wellbeing: experiencing bereavement and ill health in marginalised young people's transitions, *Sociology of Health and Illness*, 35(1): 147–61, doi:10.1111/j.1467-9566.2012.01488.x

Mackenbach, J.P., Kulhánová, I., Artnik, B., Bopp, M., Borrell, C., Clemens, T., Costa, G., Dibben, C., Kalcdiene, R., Lundberg, O. and Martikainen, P. (2016) Changes in mortality inequalities over two decades: register based study of European countries, *BMJ*, 353, i1732, doi:10.1136/bmj.i1732

MacLeavy, J. (2011) A 'new politics' of austerity, workfare and gender? The UK coalition government's welfare reform proposals, *Cambridge Journal of Regions Economy and Society*, 4(3): 355–67.

Macpherson, J. and Dobson, C. (2020) Lancashire GP warns of serious illnesses being missed in COVID-19 crisis, https://www.lancs.live/news/lancashire-news/lancashire-gp-warns-serious-illnesses-18141082; 2020

Mahase, E.J. (2020a) COVID-19: EU states report 60% rise in emergency calls about domestic violence, *BMJ*, 369: m1872.

Mahase, E.J. (2020b) COVID-19: what do we know about 'long covid'? *BMJ*, 370: m2815.

Mamelund, S.E. (1998) The diffusion of influenza in Norway during the 1918–19 pandemic, *Norwegian Journal of Epidemiology*, 8(1): 45–58.

Mamelund, S.E. (2006) A socially neutral disease? Individual social class, household wealth and mortality from Spanish influenza in two socially contrasting parishes in Kristiania 1918–19, *Social Science and Medecine*, 62: 923–40.

Manderbacka, K., Lahelma, E. and Rahkonen, O. (2001) Structural changes and social inequalities in health in Finland, 1986–1994, *Scandinavian Journal of Public Health*, 29: 41–54.

Manzo, L.K.C. and Minello, A. (2020) Mothers, childcare duties, and remote working under COVID-19 lockdown in Italy: cultivating communities of care, *Dialogues in Human Geography*, 10(2): 120–3.

Marmot, M. (2006) Introduction, in M. Marmot and R.G. Wilkinson (eds) *Social Determinants of Health*, Oxford: Oxford University Press, pp 1–5.

Marmot, M. (2010) *Fair Society Health Lives: The Marmot Review*, University College London.

Marmot, M. and Wilkinson, R.G. (eds) (2006) *Social Determinants of Health*, Oxford: Oxford University Press.

Marmot, M., Allen, J., Goldblatt, P., Boyce, T., McNeish, D. and Grady, M. (2010) *Fair Society Healthy Lives: The Marmot Review*, London: Institute of Health Equity.

Marmot, M., Allen, J., Boyce, T., Goldblatt, P. and Morrison, J. (2020) *Health Equity in England: The Marmot Review 10 Years on,* London: Institute of Health Equity, https://www.health.org. uk/publications/reports/the-marmot-review-10-years-on

Martinez, R., Lloyd-Sherlock, P., Soliz, P., Ebrahim, S., Vega, E., Ordunez, P., and McKee, M. (2020) Trends in premature avertable mortality from non-communicable diseases for 195 countries and territories, 1990–2017: a population-based study, *The Lancet Global Health*, 8(4): e511–e523.

Martins-Filho, P.R., de Souza Araújo, A.A., Quintans-Júnior, L.J. and Santana Santos, V. (2020) COVID-19 fatality rates related to social inequality in Northeast Brazil: a neighbourhood-level analysis, *Journal of Travel Medicine*, 27(7), taaa128

Martins Van Jaarsveld, G. (2020) The effects of COVID-19 among the elderly population: a case for closing the digital divide, *Frontiers in Psychiatry*, 11: 577427.

Mathias, K., Rawat, M., Philip, S. and Grills, N. (2020) 'We've got through hard times before': acute mental distress and coping among disadvantaged groups during COVID-19 lockdown in North India: a qualitative study, *International Journal for Equity in Health*, 19(1): 224.

Mattheys, K., Warren, J. and Bambra, C. (2018) 'Treading in sand': a qualitative study of the impact of austerity on inequalities in mental health, *Social Policy and Administration*, 52: 1275–89.

Matzopoulos, R., Walls, H., Cook, S. and London, L. (2020) South Africa's COVID-19 alcohol sales ban: the potential for better policy-making, *International Journal of Health Policy and Management*, 9(11): 486-7.

McCartney, G., Dickie, E., Escobar, O. and Collins, C. (2021) Health inequalities, fundamental causes and power: towards the practice of good theory, *Sociology of Health and Illness*, https://doi.org/10.1111/1467-9566.13181

McCracken, K. and Curson, P. (2003) Flu downunder: a demographic and geographic analysis of the 1919 pandemic in Sydney, Australia, in D. Killingray and H. Phillips (eds) *The Spanish Influenza Pandemic of 1918–1919: New Perspectives*, London: Routledge.

McLaughlin, M. and Rank, M. (2018) Estimating the economic cost of childhood poverty in the United States, *Social Work Research*, 42(2): 73–83.

McNamara, C.L., Balaj, M., Thomson, K.H., Eikemo, T.A., Solheim, E.F. and Bambra, C. (2017) The socioeconomic distribution of non-communicable diseases in Europe: findings from the European Social Survey (2014) special module on the social determinants of health, *European Journal of Public Health*, 27(Suppl1): 22–6.

McNamara, C.L., Balaj, M., Thomson, K.H., Eikemo, T.A. and Bambra, C. (2017) The contribution of housing and neighborhood conditions to educational inequalities in non-communicable diseases in Europe: findings from the European Social Survey (2014) special module on the social determinants of health, *European Journal of Public Health*, 27 (Suppl1): 102–6.

McQuaid, R.J., Cox, S.M.L., Ogunlana, A. and Jaworska, N. (2021) The burden of loneliness: implications of the social determinants of health during COVID-19, *Psychiatry Research*, 296: 113648.

Menachemi, N., Yiannoutsos, C.T., Dixon, B.E., Duszynski, T.J., Fadel, W.F., Wools-Kaloustian, K.K., Needleman, N.U., Box, K., Caine, V., Norwood, C. and Weaver, L. (2020) Population point prevalence of SARS-CoV-2 infection based on a statewide random sample: Indiana, April 25–29, 2020, *Morbidity and Mortality Weekly Report*, 69: 960–4, doi: http://dx.doi.org/10.15585/mmwr.mm6929e1

Miconi, D., Li, Z.Y., Frounfelker, R.L., Santavicca, T., Cénat, J.M., Venkatesh, V. and Rousseau, C. (2021) Ethno-cultural disparities in mental health during the COVID-19 pandemic: a cross-sectional study on the impact of exposure to the virus and COVID-19-related discrimination and stigma on mental health, across ethno-cultural groups in Quebec (Canada), *BJPsych Open*, 7(1): e14.

Miranda, V. (2011) *Cooking, caring and volunteering: unpaid work around the world,* OECD Social, Employment and Migration Working Papers, 116, Paris: OECD Publishing.

Mittal, S., and Singh, T. (2020) Gender-based violence during COVID-19 pandemic: a mini-review, *Frontiers in Global Women's Health*, 1: 4, https://doi.org/10.3389/fgwh.2020.00004

Moeller, H. (2013) Rising unemployment and increasing spatial health inequalities in England: further extension of the North–South divide, *Journal of Public Health*, 35(2): 313–21.

Montgomery, S.M. (1999) Unemployment, cigarette smoking, alcohol consumption and body weight in young British men, *European Journal of Public Health*, 8(1): 21–7.

Montgomery, S.M., Cook, D.G., Bartley, M.J. and Wadsworth, M.E. (1999) Unemployment pre-dates symptoms of depression and anxiety resulting in medical consultation in young men, *International Journal of Epidemiology*, 28: 95–100.

Morris, K., Beckfield, J. and Bambra, C. (2019) Who benefits from social investment? The gendered effects of employment and family policies on cardiovascular disease in Europe, *Journal of Epidemiology and Community Health*, 73: 206–13.

Morrissey, T.W. (2009) Multiple child-care arrangements and young children's behavioral outcomes. *Child Development*, 80(1): 59–76.

Muir, J. (1911) *My First Summer in the Sierra*, Boston, New York: Houghton Mifflin.

Naa Oyo, A., Kwate, C., Ji-Meng, L. and Williams, D. (2009) Inequality in obesogenic environments: fast food density in New York City, *Health & Place*, 15: 364–73.

National Center for Health Statistics (2018) Health, United States 2018, https://www.cdc.gov/nchs/data/hus/hus18.pdf#Highlights

National Records of Scotland (2020) https://www.nrscotland.gov.uk/covid19stats and https://www.bbc.co.uk/news/uk-scotland-52637581

Navarro, V., Muntaner, C., Borrell, C., Benach, J., Quiroga, A., Rodríguez-Sanz, M., Vergés, N. and Pasarín, M.I. (2006) Politics and health outcomes, *The Lancet*, 368(9540): 1033–7, doi: 10.1016/S0140-6736(06)69341-0

Neidhoefer, G., Lustig, N. and Tommasi, M. (2021) *Intergenerational transmission of lockdown consequences: prognosis of the longer-run persistence of COVID-19 in Latin America*, Working Papers 571, Society for the Study of Economic Inequality.

New American Standard Bible 2020 [1971] https://www.biblegateway.com/versions/New-American-Standard-Bible-NASB/

Nguyen, K., Glantz, S., Palmer, C. and Schmidt, L. (2020) Transferring racial/ethnic marketing strategies from tobacco to food corporations: Philip Morris and Kraft General Foods, *American Journal of Public Health*, 110: 329–36.

NHSA (Northern Health Sciences Alliance) (2020) Analysis of COVID-19 ONS Data March to May 2020, https://www.thenhsa.co.uk/app/uploads/2020/07/NHSA-COVID-REPORT-1.pdf

Niedzwiedz, C.L., Green, M.J., Benzeval, M., Campbell, D., Craig, P., Demou, E., Leyland, A., Pearce, A., Thomson, R., Whitley, E. and Katikireddi, S.V. (2020) Mental health and health behaviours before and during the COVID-19 lockdown: longitudinal analyses of the UK Household Longitudinal Study, *Journal of Epidemiology and Community Health*, 75(3): 224–31.

Niedzwiedz, C.L., Mitchell, R.J., Shortt, N.K. and Pearce, J.R. (2016) Social protection spending and inequalities in depressive symptoms across Europe, *Social Psychiatry and Psychiatric Epidemiology*, 51: 1005–14.

Nolte, E., Brand, A., Koupilová, I. and McKee, M. (2000) Neonatal and postneonatal mortality in Germany since unification, *Journal of Epidemiology and Community Health*, 54(2): 84–90.

Nolte, E., Scholz, R., Shkolnikov, V. and McKee, M. (2002) The contribution of medical care to changing life expectancy in Germany and Poland, *Social Science & Medicine*, 55(11): 1905–21.

Nurse, A. and Dunning, R. (2020) Is COVID-19 a turning point for active travel in cities? *Cities and Health*, doi: 10.1080/23748834.2020.1788769

Nyashanu, M., Pfende, F. and Ekpenyong, M.S. (2020) Triggers of mental health problems among frontline healthcare workers during the COVID-19 pandemic in private care homes and domiciliary care agencies: lived experiences of care workers in the Midlands region, UK, *Health and Social Care in the Community*, doi:10.1111/hsc.13204

O'Connor, R.C., Wetherall, K., Cleare, S., McClelland, H., Melson, A.J., Niedzwiedz, C.L., O'Carroll, R.E., O'Connor, D.B., Platt, S., Scowcroft, E. and Watson, B. (2020) Mental health and well-being during the COVID-19 pandemic: longitudinal analyses of adults in the UK COVID-19 Mental Health and Wellbeing study, *British Journal of Psychiatry*, 1–8, doi: https://doi.org/10.1192/bjp.2020.212

OECD (2015) Education at a Glance Interim Report: update of employment and educational attainment indicators, http://www.oecd.org/education/EAG-Interim-report-Chapter2.pdf

OECD (2020) Health at a Glance: Europe 2020, https://www.oecd.org/health/health-at-a-glance-europe/

Olmos, C., and Stuardo, V. (2020) Distribution of COVID-19 and tuberculosis in the metropolitan region of Chile: different diseases, similar inequalities, *Revista Médica de Chile*, 148(7): 963–9, https://dx.doi.org/10.4067/S0034-98872020000700963

ONS (Office for National Statistics) (2014) Suicides in the United Kingdom: 2012 Registrations, https://www.ons.gov.uk/peoplepopulationandcommunity/birthsdeathsandmarriages/deaths/bulletins/suicidesintheunitedkingdom/2014-02-18

ONS (2015) Inequality in healthy life expectancy at birth by national deciles of area deprivation: England, 2011 to 2013, https://www.ons.gov.uk/peoplepopulationandcommunity/healthandsocialcare/healthandlifeexpectancies/datasets/inequalityinhealthylifeexpectan cyatbirthbynationaldecilesofareadeprivationengland

ONS (2016) Adult smoking habits in the UK: 2015, https://www.ons.gov.uk/peoplepopulationandcommunity/healthandsocialcare/healthandlifeexpectancies/bulletins/adultsmokinghabitsingreatb ritain/2015

ONS (2020a) Deaths involving COVID-19 by local area and socioeconomic deprivation: deaths occurring between 1 March and 31 May 2020, https://www.ons.gov.uk/peoplepopulation andcommunity/birthsdeathsandmarriages/deaths/bulletins/ dea thsinvolvingcovid19bylocalareasanddeprivation/deathsoccurrin gbetween1marchand31may2020

ONS (2020b) Deaths involving COVID-19 by local area and socioeconomic deprivation: deaths occurring between 1 March and 31 July 2020, https://www.ons.gov.uk/peoplepopulation andcommunity/birthsdeathsandmarriages/deaths/bulletins/deaths involvingcovid19bylocalareasanddeprivation/latest

ONS (2020c) Coronavirus (COVID-19) related deaths by occupation, England and Wales: deaths registered between 9 March and 25 May 2020. https://www.ons.gov.uk/peoplepopulationandcommunity/health andsocialcare/causesofdeath/bulletins/coronavirus covid19relateddeathsbyoccupationenglandandwales/latest# overview- of-coronavirus-related-deaths-by-occupation

Orben, A., Tomova, L. and Blakemore, S-J. (2020) The effects of social deprivation on adolescent development and mental health, *The Lancet Child and Adolescent Health*, 4(8): 634–40.

O'Reilly, A. (2020) Trying to function in the unfunctionable: mothers and COVID-19, *Journal of the Motherhood Initiative for Research and Community Involvement*, 11(1): 7–24.

Palese, M. (2018) The Irish abortion referendum: how a citizens' assembly helped to break years of political deadlock, Electoral Reform Society Blog, https://www.electoral-reform.org.uk/ the-irish-abortion-referendum-how-a-citizens-assembly-helped-to-break-years-of-political-deadlock/

Palladino, L. and Karlsson, K. (2018) Towards accountable capitalism: remaking corporate law through stakeholder governance. Roosevelt Institute Issue Brief, October.

Parkes, K.S. (1997) *Understanding Contemporary Germany*, London: Taylor & Francis.

Parry, C.D. and Dewing, S. (2006) A public health approach to addressing alcohol-related crime in South Africa, *African Journal of Drug and Alcohol Studies*, 5(1): 41–56.

Parry, L.J., Asenbaum, H. and Ercan, S.A. (2020) Democracy in flux: a systemic view on the impact of COVID-19, *Transforming Government: People, Process and Policy*, https://doi.org/10.1108/ TG-09-2020-0269

Patz, J.A., Epstein, P.R., Burke, T.A. and Balbus, J.M. (1996) Global climate change and emerging infectious diseases, *JAMA*, 275(3): 217–23.

Pearce, D.C., Pallaghy, P.K., McCaw, J.M., McVernon J. and Mathews, J.D. (2011) Understanding mortality in the 1918–1919 influenza pandemic in England and Wales, *Influenza and Other Respiratory Viruses*, 5(2): 89–98.

Pearce, J., Dorling, D., Wheeler, B., Barnett, R. and Rigby, J. (2006) Geographical inequalities in health in New Zealand, 1980–2001: the gap widens, *Australian and New Zealand Journal of Public Health*, 30(5): 461–6.

Pellegrini, M., Ponzo, V., Rosato, R., Scumaci, E., Goitre, I., Benso, A., Belcastro, S., Crespi, C., De Michieli, F., Ghigo, E. and Broglio, F. (2020) Changes in weight and nutritional habits in adults with obesity during the 'lockdown' period caused by the COVID-19 virus emergency, *Nutrients*, 12(7): 2016.

Pensiero, N., Kelly, A. and Bokhove, C. (2020) *Learning Inequalities during the COVID-19 Pandemic: How Families Cope with Home-schooling*, Southampton: University of Southampton.

Peretti-Watel, P., Seror, V., Cortaredona, S., Launay, O., Raude, J., Verger, P., Beck, F., Legleye, S., L'Haridon, O. and Ward, J. (2021) Attitudes about COVID-19 lockdown among general population, France, March 2020, *Emerging Infectious Diseases*, 27(1): 301–3.

Pérez-González, L. (2020) The government is following the science: why is the translation of evidence into policy generating so much controversy? LSE Blog, https://blogs.lse.ac.uk/impactofsocialsciences/2020/11/12/the-government-is-following-the-science-why-is-the-translation-of-evidence-into-policy-generating-so-much-controversy/

Petersen, C.B., Mortensen, L.H., Morgen, C.S., Madsen, M., Schnor, O., Arntzen, A., Gissler, M., Cnattingius, S. and Nybo Andersen., A. (2009) Socio-economic inequality in preterm birth: a comparative study of the Nordic countries from 1981 to 2000, *Paediatric and Perinatal Epidemiology*, 23(1): 66–75.

Pew Research Center (2020) Unemployment rose higher in three months of COVID-19 than it did in two years of the Great Recession, https://www.pewresearch.org/fact-tank/2020/06/11/unemployment-rose-higher-in-three-months-of-covid-19-than-it-did-in-two-years-of-the-great-recession/ (Accessed 4 November 2020)

PHE (Public Health England) (2020) COVID-19: review of disparities in risks and outcomes, https://www.gov.uk/government/publications/covid-19-review-of-disparities-in-risks-and-outcomes (Accessed 2 October 2020)

Pierce, M., Hope, H., Ford, T., Hatch, S., Hotopf, M., John, A., Kontopantelis, E., Webb, R., Wessely, S., McManus, S. and Abel, K.M. (2020) Mental health before and during the COVID-19 pandemic: a longitudinal probability sample survey of the UK population, *The Lancet Psychiatry*, 7(10): 883–92.

Pierson, P. (2000) Increasing returns, path dependence, and the study of politics, *American Political Science Review*, 94(2): 251–67, doi:10.2307/2586011

Pierson, P. (2011) *Politics in Time: History, Institutions, and Social Analysis*, Princeton, NJ: Princeton University Press.

Pleyers, G. (2020) The pandemic is a battlefield: social movements in the COVID-19 lockdown, *Journal of Civil Society*, 16(4): 1–18.

Popham, F., Dibben, C. and Bambra, C. (2013) Are inequalities in mortality really not the smallest in the Scandinavian welfare states? A comparative total inequality analysis of life expectancy in 37 countries, *Journal of Epidemiology and Community Health*, 67: 412–18.

Prati, G., Pietrantoni, L. and Zani, B. (2011) Compliance with recommendations for pandemic influenza H1N1 2009: the role of trust and personal beliefs, *Health Education Research*, 26(5): 761–9.

Proto, E. and Quintana-Domeque, C. (2021) COVID-19 and mental health deterioration by ethnicity and gender in the UK, *PLOS ONE*, 16(1): e0244419.

Public Health Agency of Sweden, (2020) Demografisk beskrivning av bekräftade COVID-19 fall i Sverige 13 mars-7 maj 2020: Folkhälsomyndigheten, Public Health Agency of Sweden, http://www.folkhalsomyndigheten.se/publicerat-material/publikationsarkiv/d/demografisk-beskrivning-av-bekraftade-covid-19-fall-i-sverige-13-mars-7-maj-2020/ (Accessed 14 January 2021)

Purtle, J. (2020) COVID-19 and mental health equity in the United States, *Social Psychiatry and Psychiatric Epidemiology*, 55(8): 969–71.

Qiu, J., Shen, B., Zhao, M., Wang, Z., Xie, B. and Xu, Y. (2020) A nationwide survey of psychological distress among Chinese people in the COVID-19 epidemic: implications and policy recommendations, *General Psychiatry*, 33(2): e100213.

Qureshi, K., Hill, S., Meer, N. and Kasstan, B. (2020) COVID-19 and BAME inequalities: the problem of institutional racism, Centre for Health and the Public Interest Blog, https://chpi.org.uk/blog/covid-19-and-bame-inequalities-the-problem-of-institutional-racism/

Reeves, Richard (2017) *Dream Hoarders: The Dangerous Separation of the American Upper Middle Class.* Washington, DC: Brookings Institute Press.

Registrar-General (1920) *Supplement to the Eighty-First Annual Report of the Registrar-General: Report on the mortality from influenza in England and Wales during the epidemic of 1918–19*, London: HMSO.

Reid, M. (2011) Behind the 'Glasgow Effect', *Bulletin of the World Health Organization*, 89(10): 706–7.

Reny, T.T. and Barreto, M.A. (2020) Xenophobia in the time of pandemic: othering, anti-Asian attitudes, and COVID-19, *Politics, Groups, and Identities*, Advanced Online Access: 1–24, https://doi.org/10.1080/21565503.2020.1769693

Rice, G. and Bryder, L. (2005) *Black November: The 1918 Influenza Pandemic in New Zealand*, Christchurch: Canterbury University Press.

Roberts, D. (2011) *Fatal Invention: How Science, Politics, and Big Business Re-Create Race in the Twenty-First Century*, New York: New Press.

Robinson, T., Brown, H., Norman, P., Barr, B., Fraser, L. and Bambra, C. (2019) Investigating the impact of New Labour's English health inequalities strategy on geographical inequalities in infant mortality: a time trend analysis, *Journal of Epidemiology and Community Health*, 73: 564–8, doi:10.1136/jech-2018-211679

Rodríguez-Urrego, D. and Rodríguez-Urrego, L. (2020) Air quality during the COVID-19: PM2.5 analysis in the 50 most polluted capital cities in the world, *Environmental Pollution*, 266(1): 115042. https://doi.org/10.1016/j.envpol.2020.115042

Roesch, E., Amin, A., Gupta, J. and García-Moreno, C. (2020) Violence against women during COVID-19 pandemic restrictions, *BMJ*, 369, m1712.

Roncon, L., Zuin, M., Rigatelli, G. and Zuliani, G. (2020) Diabetic patients with COVID-19 infection are at higher risk of ICU admission and poor short-term outcome, *Journal of Clinical Virology*, 127: 104354, doi:10.1016/j. jcv.2020.104354

Ruhm, C.J. (2000) Are recessions good for your health?, *Quarterly Journal of Economics*, 115(2): 617–50.

Rutter, P.D., Mytton, O.T., Mak, M. and Donaldson, L.J. (2012) Socio-economic disparities in mortality due to pandemic influenza in England, *International Journal of Public Health*, 57, 745–50.

Ryan, P.G., Maclean, K. and Weideman, E.A. (2020) The impact of the COVID-19 lockdown on urban street litter in South Africa, *Environmental Processes*, 7(4): 1303–12.

Sabatello, M., Scroggins, M.J., Goto, G., Santiago, A., McCormick, A., Morris, K.J., Daulton, C.R., Easter, C.L. and Darien, G. (2020) Structural racism in the COVID-19 pandemic: moving forward, *American Journal of Bioethics*, doi: 10.1080/15265161.2020.1851808

Sapey, E., Gallier, S., Mainey, C., Nightingale, P., McNulty, D., Crothers, H., Evison, F., Reeves, K., Pagano, D., Denniston, A.K. and Nirantharakumar, K. (2020) Ethnicity and risk of death in patients hospitalised for COVID-19 infection: an observational cohort study in an urban catchment area, *BMJ Open Respiratory Research*, doi: 10.1136/bmjresp-2020-000644

Scheidel, W. (2017) *The Great Leveler: Violence and the History Of Inequality from the Stone Age to the Twenty-First Century*, Princeton, NJ: Princeton University Press

Schrecker, T. and Bambra., C. (2015) *How Politics Makes Us Sick: Neoliberal Epidemics*, London: Palgrave Macmillan.

Scott-Samuel, A., Bambra, C., Collins, C., Hunter, D., McCartney, G. and Smith, K. (2014) The impact of Thatcherism on health and well-being in Britain, *International Journal of Health Services*, 44(1): 53–71.

Scruggs, L. and Allan, J.P. (2006) The material consequences of welfare states: benefit generosity and absolute poverty in 16 OECD countries, *Comparative Political Studies*, 39(7): 880–904, doi:10.1177/0010414005281935

Segerstrom, S.C. and Miller, G.E. (2004) Psychological stress and the human immune system: a meta-analytic study of 30 years of inquiry, *Psychological Bulletin*, 130(4): 601–30, doi:10.1037/0033-2909.130.4.601

Sequoia (2020) The Black Swan of 2020, Sequoia Capital Publication, Medium https://medium.com/sequoia-capital/coronavirus-the-black-swan-of-2020-7c72bdeb9753 (Accessed 12 January 2021)

Shoari, N., Ezzati, M., Baumgartner, J., Malacarne, D. and Fecht, D. (2020) Accessibility and allocation of public parks and gardens in England and Wales: a COVID-19 social distancing perspective, *PLOS ONE*, 15(10): e0241102.

Sidor, A. and Rzymski, P. (2020) Dietary choices and habits during COVID-19 lockdown: experience from Poland, *Nutrients*, 12(6): 1657.

Sigurdsson, E.L., Blondal, A.B., Jonsson, J.S., Tomasdottir, M.O., Hrafnkelsson, H., Linnet, K. and Sigurdsson, J.A. (2020) How primary healthcare in Iceland swiftly changed its strategy in response to the COVID-19 pandemic, *BMJ Open*, 10(12): e043151, doi:10.1136/bmjopen-2020-043151

Simonnet, A., Chetboun, M., Poissy, J., Raverdy, V., Noulette, J., Duhamel, A., Labreuche, J., Mathieu, D., Pattou, F., Jourdain, M. and LICORN and the Lille COVID-19 and Obesity Study Group (2020) High prevalence of obesity in severe acute respiratory syndrome coronavirus-2 (SARS-CoV-2) requiring invasive mechanical ventilation, *Obesity*, 28(7): 1195–9, doi:10.1002/oby.22831.

Singer, M. (2000) A dose of drugs, a touch of violence, a case of AIDS: conceptualizing the SAVA syndemic, *Free Inquiry in Creative Sociology*, 28: 13–24.

Singer, M. (2009) *Introduction to Syndemics: A Systems Approach to Public and Community Health,* San Francisco, CA: Jossey-Bass.

Sintomer, Y., Herzberg, C. and Röcke, A. (2008) Participatory budgeting in Europe: potentials and challenges, *International Journal of Urban and Regional Research*, 32(1): 164–78.

SkyNews (2020) Virus does not discriminate claims Gove [Conservative government Minister for the Cabinet Office, UK], 27 March, https://news.sky.com/video/coronavirus-virus-does-not-discriminate-gove-11964771 (Accessed 22 April 2020)

Slater, S.J., Christiana, R.W. and Gustat, J. (2020) Recommendations for keeping parks and green space accessible for mental and physical health during COVID-19 and other pandemics, *Preventing Chronic Disease*, 17: 200204, doi:http://dx.doi.org/10.5888/pcd17.200204

Smith, K.E. and Anderson, R. (2018) Understanding lay perspectives on socioeconomic health inequalities in Britain: a meta-ethnography, *Sociology of Health and Illness*, 40(1): 146–70.

Soga, M., Evans, M.J., Tsuchiya, K. and Fukano, Y. (2020) A room with a green view: the importance of nearby nature for mental health during the COVID-19 pandemic, *Ecological Applications*, 31(2): e02248, 10.1002/eap.2248

Steyn, N., Binny, R.N., Hannah, K., Hendy, S., James, A., Kukutai, T., Lustig, A., McLeod, M., Plank, M.J., Ridings, K. and Sporle, A. (2020) Estimated inequities in COVID-19 infection fatality rates by ethnicity for Aotearoa New Zealand, https://doi.org/10.1101/2020.04.20.20073437

Stroebe, M., Schut, H. and Stroebe, W. (2007) Health outcomes of bereavement, *The Lancet*, 370(9603): 1960–73.

Struwig, J., Roberts, B.J. and Gordon, S.L. (2020) Dark cloud with a silver lining? The prospect of a rise in material values or a post-material turn in post-pandemic South Africa, *International Journal of Sociology*, doi: 10.1080/00207659.2020.1826106

Stuckler, D. and Basu, S. (2013) *The Body Economic: Why Austerity Kills*, London: Allan Lane.

Stuckler, D., Basu, S., Suhrcke, M., Coutts, A. and McKee, M. (2009) The public health effect of economic crises and alternative policy responses in Europe: an empirical analysis, *The Lancet*, 374: 315–23.

Summers, J.A., Stanley, J., Baker, M.G. and Wilson, N. (2014) Risk factors for death from pandemic influenza in 1918–1919: a case-control study, *Influenza and Other Respiratory Viruses*, 8(3): 329–38, https://doi.org/10.1111/irv.12228

Swedo, E., Idaikkadar, N., Leemis, R., Dias, T., Radhakrishnan, L., Stein, Z., Chen, M., Agathis, N. and Holland, K. (2020) Trends in US emergency department visits related to suspected or confirmed child abuse and neglect among children and adolescents aged <18 years before and during the COVID-19 pandemic: United States, January 2019–September 2020, *Morbidity and Mortality Weekly Report*, 69(49): 1841–7.

Sydenstricker, E. (2006 [1931]) The incidence of influenza among persons of different economic status during the epidemic of 1918, *Public Health Reports*, 121(Suppl1): 191–204.

Sylvers, E. (2021) COVID-19 hit hardest where financial crisis led to health-care cuts, *Wall Street Journal*, 11 January, https://www.wsj.com/articles/covid-19-hit-hardest-where-financial-crisis-led-to-health-care-cuts-11610372026 (Accessed 12 January 2021)

Taleb, N.N. (2010) *The Black Swan: The Impact of the Highly Improbable*, 2nd edn, New York: Random House Trade Paperbacks.

Tam, K., Yousey-Hindes, K. and Hadler, L. (2014) Influenza-related hospitalization of adults associated with low census tract socioeconomic status and female sex in New Haven County, Connecticut, 2007–2011, *Influenza and other Respiratory Viruses*, 8: 274–81, doi:10.1111/irv.12231

Tapia Granados, J.A. (2005) Increasing mortality during the expansions of the US economy, 1900–1996, *International Journal of Epidemiology*, 34: 1194–1202.

Taylor-Robinson, D., Lai, E., Wickham, S., Rose, T., Bambra, C., Whitehead, M. and Barr, B. (2019) Assessing the impact of rising child poverty on the unprecedented rise in infant mortality in England, 2000–2017: time trend analysis, *BMJ Open*, 9: e029424, doi: 10.1136/bmjopen-2019-029424

Teachout, M. and Zipfel C. (2020) The economic impact of COVID-19 lockdowns in subSaharan Africa, Policy Brief, International Growth Centre, https://www.theigc.org/wp-content/uploads/2020/05/Teachout-and-Zipfel-2020-policy-brief-.pdf

Thelen, K.A. (2014) *Varieties of Liberalization and the New Politics of Social Solidarity*. Cambridge: Cambridge University Press.

Thirlway, F. (2020) Explaining the social gradient in smoking and cessation: the peril and promise of social mobility, *Sociology of Health and Illness*, 42: 565–78.

Thomas, E. and Whitehead, L. (2020) Using the flexibility of civil society to overcome COVID-19: the local knowledge and adaptability of civil society organizations are proving valuable during the ongoing pandemic, *Asian Development Blog*, https://blogs.adb.org/blog/using-flexibility-civil-society-overcome-covid-19

Thomas, E.Y., Anurudran, A., Robb, K. and Burke, T.F. (2020) Spotlight on child abuse and neglect response in the time of COVID-19, *The Lancet Public Health*, 5(7): e371, https://doi.org/10.1016/S2468-2667(20)30143-2

Thucydides (431BC) *The Peloponnesian War*, https://www.gutenberg.org/files/7142/7142-h/7142-h.htm

Todd, A., Copeland, A., Husband, A., Kasim, A. and Bambra, C. (2015) Access all areas? An area-level analysis of the relationship between community pharmacy and primary care distribution, urbanity and social deprivation in England, *BMJ Open*, 5: e007328, http://dx.doi.org/10.1136/bmjopen-2014-007328

Tyler, I. (2020) *Stigma: The Machinery of Inequality*, London: Zed Books.

UBS (2020) Billionaires insights 2020, https://www.pwc.ch/en/publications/2020/UBS-PwC-Billionaires-Report-2020.pdf

Ugolini, F., Massetti, L., Calaza-Martínez, P., Cariñanos, P., Dobbs, C., Ostoić, S.K., Marin, A.M., Pearlmutter, D., Saaroni, H., Šaulienė, I. and Simoneti, M. (2020) Effects of the COVID-19 pandemic on the use and perceptions of urban green space: an international exploratory study, *Urban Forestry and Urban Greening*, 56: 126888.

United Nations (2020a) UN Secretary-General's policy brief: the impact of COVID-19 on women, https://www.unwomen.org/en/digital-library/publications/2020/04: UN; 2020.

United Nations (2020b) UN Working to Avert Dual Crises as COVID-19 Hits Hunger Hotspots, https://www.un.org/en/un-coronavirus-communications-team/un-working-avert-dual-crises-covid-19-hits-hunger-hotspots

Usher, K., Bhullar, N., Durkin, J., Gyamfi, N. and Jackson, D. (2020) Family violence and COVID-19: increased vulnerability and reduced options for support, *International Journal of Mental Health Nursing*, 29(4): 549–52.

Valkonen, T., Martikainen, P., Jalovaara, M., Koskinen, S., Martelin, T. and Makela, P. (2000) Changes in socioeconomic inequalities in mortality during an economic boom and recession among middle-aged men and women in Finland, *European Journal of Public Health*, 10: 274–80.

Van Tilburg, T.G., Steinmetz, S., Stolte, E., van der Roest, H. and de Vries, D.H. (2020) Loneliness and mental health during the COVID-19 pandemic: a study among Dutch older adults, *Journals of Gerontology: Series B*, doi: 10.1093/geronb/gbaa111

Venter, Z.S., Barton, D.N., Gundersen, V., Figari, H. and Nowell, M. (2020) Urban nature in a time of crisis: recreational use of green space increases during the COVID-19 outbreak in Oslo, Norway, *Environmental Research Letters*, 15(10): 104075.

Vizard, P. and Obolenskaya, P. (2015) The Coalition's record on health: policy, spending and outcomes 2010–2015, *Social Policy in a Cold Climate*, Working Paper 16, RePEc:cep:spccwp:16

Walker, A. and Wong, C. (eds) (2005) East Asian welfare regimes in transition: from Confucianism to globalisation, 1st ed, Bristol: Bristol University Press, doi:10.2307/j.ctt9qgm39

Walker, R., Kyomuhendo, G., Bantebya, C. and Choudry, E. (2013) Poverty in global perspective: is shame a common denominator?, *Journal of Social Policy*, 42: 215–33.

Walkerdine, V. (2010) Communal beingness and affect: an exploration of trauma in an ex-industrial community, *Body and Society*, 16: 91–116.

Walsh, D., McCartney, G., Minton, J., Parkinson, J., Shipton, D. and Whyte, B. (2020) Changing mortality trends in countries and cities of the UK: a population-based trend analysis, *BMJ Open*, 10(11): e038135.

Whitehead, M. (2007) A typology of actions to tackle social inequalities in health, *Journal of Epidemiology and Community Health*, 61: 473–8.

Whitehead, M. and Popay, J. (2010) Swimming upstream? Taking action on the social determinants of health inequalities, *Social Science and Medicine*, 71(7): 1234–6.

Whitehead, M., Pennington, A., Orton, L., Nayak, S., Petticrew, M., Sowden, A. and White, M. (2016) How could differences in 'control over destiny' lead to socio-economic inequalities in health? A synthesis of theories and pathways in the living environment, *Health and Place*, 39: 51–61.

WHO (World Health Organization) (2008) *Closing the Gap in a Generation: Health Equity Through Action on the Social Determinants of Health*, Geneva: World Health Organisation, https://www.who. int/social_determinants/thecommission/finalreport/en/

Wilkinson, R. and Pickett, K. (2009) *The Spirit Level: Why More Equal Societies Almost Always Do Better*, London: Allen Lane.

Women's Aid (2020) A perfect storm: the impact of the covid-19 pandemic on domestic abuse survivors and the services supporting them, https://www.womensaid.org.uk/wp-content/uploads/2020/08/A-Perfect-Storm-August-2020-1.pdf)

Wong, C.A., Ming, D., Maslow, G. and Gifford, E.J. (2020) Mitigating the impacts of the COVID-19 pandemic response on at-risk children, *Paediatrics*, 146(1): e20200973.

Wood, L., Baumler, E., Schrag, R.V., Guillot-Wright, S., Hairston, D., Temple, J. and Torres, E. (2021) 'Don't know where to go for help': safety and economic needs among violence survivors during the COVID-19 pandemic, *Journal of Family Violence*, https://doi. org/10.1007/s10896-020-00240-7

Wright, J. (2021) Coronavirus doctor's diary: Karen caught COVID: and took it home, https://www.bbc.co.uk/news/stories-55682405

Wu, X., Lu, Y., Zhou, S., Chen, L. and Xu, B. (2016) Impact of climate change on human infectious diseases: empirical evidence and human adaptation, *Environment International*, 86:14–23, doi:10.1016/j.envint.2015.09.007

Wucker, M. (2016) *The Gray Rhino: How to Recognize and Act on the Obvious Dangers We Ignore*, New York: St. Martin's Press.

Yakubovich, A.R., Stöckl, H., Murray, J., Melendez-Torres, G.J., Steinert, J.I., Glavin, C.E.Y. and Humphreys, D.K. (2018) Risk and protective factors for intimate partner violence against women: systematic review and meta-analyses of prospective–longitudinal studies, *American Journal of Public Health*, 108(7): e1-e11.

Zadnik, V., Mihor, A., Tomsic, S., Zagar, T., Bric, N., Lokar, K. and Oblak, I. (2020) Impact of COVID-19 on cancer diagnosis and management in Slovenia: preliminary results, *Radiology and Oncology*, 54(3): 329–34.

Zavras, D., Tsiantou, V., Pavi, E., Mylona, K. and Kyriopoulos, J. (2013) Impact of economic crisis and other demographic and socio-economic factors on self-rated health in Greece, *European Journal of Public Health*, 23(2): 206–10.

Zhang, H. (2020) The influence of the ongoing COVID-19 pandemic on family violence in China, *Journal of Family Violence*, https://doi.org/10.1007/s10896-020-00196-8

Index